GMO FREE

Exposing the Hazards of Biotechnology to Ensure the Integrity of Our Food Supply

Independent Science Panel
Mae-Wan Ho and Lim Li Ching

with contributions from

Joe Cummins, Malcolm Hooper, Miguel Altieri,
Peter Rosset, Arpad Pusztai, Stanley Ewen,
Michel Pimbert, Peter Saunders, Edward Goldsmith,
David Quist, Eva Novotny, Vyvyan Howard, Brian Jones
and others on the Panel

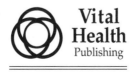
Vital Health Publishing

Ridgefield, CT

GMO Free: Exposing the Hazards of Biotechnology
to Ensure the Integrity of Our Food Supply

Book Design: interior, Cathy Lombardi; cover, On The Dot Designs

Published by: Vital Health Publishing
               P.O. Box 152
               Ridgefield, CT 06877
               Web site: www.vitalhealthbooks.com
               E-mail: info@vitalhealthbooks.com
               Phone: 203-894-1882
               Orders: 1-877-VIT-BOOK

Originally published by: Institute of Science in Society
                          PO Box 32097
                          London NW1 0XR, UK
                          &
                          Third World Network
                          121-S Jalan Utama
                          10450 Penang, Malaysia

Printed in the United States of America
ISBN: 1-890612-37-5

Preface

Members of the Independent Science Panel (ISP) on GM have had the opportunity to review extensive scientific and other evidence on genetic engineering over the past decades. Many are among the more than 600 scientists from 72 countries who have signed an "Open Letter from World Scientists to All Governments" [1], initiated in 1999, which called for a moratorium on the environmental release of genetically modified organisms (GMOs), a ban on patents on living processes, organisms, seeds, cell lines and genes, and a comprehensive public enquiry into the future of agriculture and food security.

Scientific and other developments since 1999 have confirmed our concerns over the safety of genetic engineering, genetically modified (GM) crops and food security. At the same time, the successes and benefits of the different forms of sustainable agriculture are undeniable. The evidence, now assembled, makes a strong case for a worldwide ban on all environmental release of GM crops to make way for a comprehensive shift to agroecology, sustainable agriculture and organic farming.

The evidence on why GM crops are not a viable option for a sustainable future is presented in Parts 1 and 2, while Part 3 presents evidence on the successes and benefits of sustainable agricultural practices.

Note

This Report is a summary of a vast amount of literature. We have included as much of the primary sources as possible, but many of the papers cited in the list of references are themselves extensive reviews of scientific and other literature, submitted to various national and international bodies that have called for evidence.

In producing the ISP Report, ISP members are responsible for those areas where they have specific competence, while giving overall endorsement to the report as a whole. Each ISP member also recognizes the expertise and authority of other ISP members in those areas where they themselves do not have specific competence.

Contents

Executive Summary

Why GM Free?

1. GM crops failed to deliver promised benefits

The consistent finding from independent research and on-farm surveys since 1999 is that genetically modified (GM) crops have failed to deliver the promised benefits of significantly increasing yields or reducing herbicide and pesticide use. GM crops have cost the United States (US) an estimated $12 billion in farm subsidies, lost sales and product recalls due to transgenic contamination. Massive failures in insect-resistant Bt cotton of up to 100% were reported in India.

Biotech corporations have suffered rapid decline since 2000, and investment advisors forecast no future for the agricultural sector. Meanwhile, worldwide resistance to GM reached a climax when, in 2002, Zambia refused GM maize (corn) in food aid despite the threat of famine.

2. GM crops posing escalating problems on the farm

The instability of transgenic lines has plagued the industry from the beginning, and this may be responsible for a string of major crop failures. A review in 1994 stated, "While there are some examples of plants which show stable expression of a transgene these may prove to be the exceptions to the rule. In an informal survey of over 30 companies involved in the commercialization of transgenic crop plants . . . almost all of the respondents indicated that they had observed some level of transgene inaction. Many respondents indicated that most cases of transgene inactivation never reach the literature."

Triple herbicide-tolerant oilseed rape (canola) volunteers* that have combined transgenic and nontransgenic traits are now widespread in Canada. Similar multiple herbicide-tolerant volunteers and weeds have emerged in the US. In the US, glyphosate-tolerant weeds are plaguing GM cotton and soya fields, and atrazine, one of the most toxic herbicides, has had to be used with glufosinate-tolerant GM maize.

Bt biopesticide traits are simultaneously threatening to create superweeds and Bt-resistant pests.

*Volunteers are plants germinated from the seeds of crops previously grown in the same fields, which are subsequently considered to be weeds.

3. Extensive transgenic contamination unavoidable

Extensive transgenic contamination has occurred in maize landraces* growing in remote regions in Mexico despite an official moratorium that has been in place since 1998. High levels of contamination have since been found in Canada. In a test of 33 samples of certified canola (oilseed rape) seed stocks, 32 were found to be contaminated.

New research shows that transgenic pollen, wind-blown and deposited elsewhere, or fallen directly to the ground, is a major source of transgenic contamination. Contamination is generally acknowledged to be unavoidable, hence *there can be no coexistence of transgenic and nontransgenic crops.*

4. GM crops not safe

Contrary to the claims of proponents, GM crops have not been proven safe. The regulatory framework was fatally flawed from the start. It was based on an antiprecautionary approach designed to expedite product approval at the expense of safety considerations.

The principle of "substantial equivalence," on which risk assessment is based, is intended to be vague and ill-defined, thereby giving companies complete licence in claiming transgenic products "substantially equivalent" to nontransgenic products, and hence "safe."

5. GM food raises serious safety concerns

There have been very few credible studies on GM food safety. Nevertheless, the available findings already give cause for concern. In the still only systematic investigation on GM food ever carried out in the world, "growth factor-like" effects were found in the stomach and small intestine of young rats that were not fully accounted for by the transgene product, and were hence attributable to the transgenic process or the transgenic construct, *and may hence be general to all GM food.*

There have been at least two other, more limited, studies that also raised serious safety concerns.

6. Dangerous gene products are incorporated into crops

Bt proteins, incorporated into 25% of all transgenic crops worldwide, have been found harmful to a range of nontarget insects. Some of them are also potent immunogens and allergens. A team of scientists has cautioned against releasing Bt crops for human use.

* Landraces are varieties of species found in local areas that are specifically adapted to grow in those areas.

Food crops are increasingly used to produce pharmaceuticals and drugs, including cytokines known to suppress the immune system, induce sickness and central nervous system toxicity; interferon alpha, reported to cause dementia, neurotoxicity and mood and cognitive side effects; vaccines; and viral sequences such as the "spike" protein gene of the pig corona virus, in the same family as the SARS virus linked to the current epidemic. The glycoprotein gene *gp120* of the AIDS virus HIV-1, incorporated into GM maize as a "cheap, edible oral vaccine," serves as yet another biological time-bomb, as it can interfere with the immune system and recombine with viruses and bacteria to generate new and unpredictable pathogens.

7. Terminator crops spread male sterility

Crops engineered with "suicide" genes for male sterility have been promoted as a means of "containing," (i.e., preventing the spread of transgenes). In reality, the hybrid crops sold to farmers spread both male sterile suicide genes as well as herbicide-tolerance genes *via* *pollen*.

8. Broad-spectrum herbicides highly toxic to humans and other species

Glufosinate ammonium and glyphosate are used with the herbicide-tolerant transgenic crops that currently account for 75% of all transgenic crops worldwide. Both are systemic metabolic poisons expected to have a wide range of harmful effects, which have been confirmed.

Glufosinate ammonium is linked to neurological, respiratory, gastrointestinal and hematological toxicities, and birth defects in humans and mammals. It is toxic to butterflies and a number of beneficial insects, also to the larvae of clams and oysters, *Daphnia* and some freshwater fish, especially the rainbow trout. It inhibits beneficial soil bacteria and fungi, especially those that fix nitrogen.

Glyphosate is the most frequent cause of complaints and poisoning in the UK. Disturbances of many body functions have been reported after exposures at normal use levels. Glyphosate exposure nearly doubled the risk of late spontaneous abortion, and children born to users of glyphosate had elevated neurobehavioral defects. Glyphosate caused retarded development of the fetal skeleton in laboratory rats. Glyphosate inhibits the synthesis of steroids, and is genotoxic in mammals, fish and frogs. Field-dose exposure of earthworms caused at least 50 percent mortality and significant intestinal damage among surviving worms. Roundup™ caused cell division dysfunction that may be linked to human cancers.

The known effects of both glufosinate and glyphosate are sufficiently serious for all further uses of the herbicides to be halted.

9. Genetic engineering creates superviruses
By far the most insidious dangers of genetic engineering are inherent to the process itself, which greatly enhances the scope and probability of horizontal gene transfer and recombination, the main route to creating viruses and bacteria that cause disease epidemics. This was highlighted in 2001 by the "accidental" creation of a killer mouse virus in the course of an apparently innocent genetic engineering experiment.

Newer techniques, such as DNA shuffling, are allowing geneticists to create, in a matter of minutes in the laboratory, millions of recombinant viruses that have never existed in billions of years of evolution.

Disease-causing viruses and bacteria and their genetic material are the predominant materials and tools for genetic engineering, as much as for the intentional creation of bioweapons.

10. Transgenic DNA in food taken up by bacteria in the human gut
There is already experimental evidence that transgenic DNA from plants has been taken up by bacteria in the soil and in the gut of human volunteers. Antibiotic-resistance marker genes can spread from transgenic food to pathogenic bacteria, making infections very difficult to treat.

11. Transgenic DNA and cancer
Transgenic DNA is known to survive digestion in the gut and to jump into the genome of mammalian cells, raising the possibility for triggering cancer.

The possibility cannot be excluded that feeding GM products such as maize to animals also carries risks, not just for the animals but also for human beings consuming the animal products.

12. CaMV 35S promoter increases horizontal gene transfer
Evidence suggests that transgenic constructs with the CaMV 35S promoter might be especially unstable and prone to horizontal gene transfer and recombination, with all the attendant hazards: gene mutations due to random insertion, cancer, reactivation of dormant viruses and generation of new viruses. This promoter is present in most GM crops being grown commercially today.

13. A history of misrepresentation and suppression of scientific evidence

There has been a history of misrepresentation and suppression of scientific evidence, especially on horizontal gene transfer. Key experiments failed to be performed, or were performed badly and then misrepresented. Many experiments were not followed up, including investigations on whether the CaMV 35S promoter is responsible for the "growth factor-like" effects observed in young rats fed GM potatoes.

In conclusion, GM crops have failed to deliver the promised benefits and are posing escalating problems on the farm. Transgenic contamination is now widely acknowledged to be unavoidable, and hence there can be no coexistence of GM and non-GM agriculture. Most important of all, GM crops have not been proven safe. On the contrary, sufficient evidence has emerged to raise serious safety concerns that, if ignored, could result in irreversible damage to health and the environment. GM crops should be firmly rejected now.

Why Sustainable Agriculture?

1. Higher productivity and yields, especially in the Third World

Some 8.98 million farmers have adopted sustainable agriculture practices on 28.92 million hectares in Asia, Latin America and Africa. Reliable data from 89 projects show higher productivity and yields: 50–100% increase in yield for rain-fed crops, and 5–10% for irrigated crops. Top successes include Burkina Faso, which turned a cereal deficit of 644 kg per year into an annual surplus of 153 kg; Ethiopia, where 12,500 households enjoyed a 60% increase in crop yields; and Honduras and Guatemala, where 45,000 families increased yields from 400–600 kg/ha to 2000–2500 kg/ha.

Long-term studies in industrialized countries show yields for organic agriculture are comparable to conventional agriculture, and sometimes higher.

2. Better soils

Sustainable agricultural practices tend to reduce soil erosion, as well as improve soil physical structure and water-holding capacity, which are crucial in averting crop failures during periods of drought.

Soil fertility is maintained or increased by various sustainable agriculture practices. Studies show that soil organic matter and nitrogen levels are higher in organic than in conventional fields.

Biological activity has also been found to be higher in organic soils. There are more earthworms, arthropods, mycorrhizal and other fungi, and microorganisms, all of which are beneficial for nutrient recycling and suppression of disease.

3. Cleaner environment

There is little or no polluting chemical input with sustainable agriculture. Moreover, research suggests that less nitrate and phosphorus are leached to groundwater from organic soils.

Better water infiltration rates are found in organic systems. Therefore, they are less prone to erosion and less likely to contribute to water pollution from surface runoff.

4. Reduced pesticides and no increase in pests

Organic farming prohibits routine pesticide application. Integrated pest management has cut the number of pesticide sprays in Vietnam from 3.4 to 1.0 per season, in Sri Lanka from 2.9 to 0.5 per season, and in Indonesia from 2.9 to 1.1 per season.

Research showed no increase in crop losses due to pest damage, despite the withdrawal of synthetic insecticides in Californian tomato production.

Pest control is achievable without pesticides, reversing crop losses, as for example, by using "trap crops" to attract stem borer, a major pest in East Africa. Other benefits of avoiding pesticides arise from utilizing the complex interrelationships between species in an ecosystem.

5. Supporting biodiversity and using diversity

Sustainable agriculture promotes agricultural biodiversity, which is crucial for food security and rural livelihoods. Organic farming can also support much greater biodiversity, benefiting species that have significantly declined.

Biodiverse systems are more productive than monocultures. Integrated farming systems in Cuba are 1.45 to 2.82 times more productive than monocultures. Thousands of Chinese rice farmers have doubled yields and nearly eliminated the most devastating disease simply by mixed planting of two varieties.

Soil biodiversity is enhanced by organic practices, bringing beneficial effects such as recovery and rehabilitation of degraded soils, improved soil structure and water infiltration.

6. Environmentally and economically sustainable

Research on apple production systems ranked the organic system first in environmental and economic sustainability, the integrated system second and the conventional system last. Organic apples were most profitable due to price premiums, quicker investment return and fast recovery of costs.

A Europe-wide study showed that organic farming performs better than conventional farming in the majority of environmental indicators. A review by the Food and Agriculture Organization of the United Nations (FAO) concluded that well-managed organic agriculture leads to more favorable conditions at all environmental levels.

7. Ameliorating climate change by reducing direct and indirect energy use

Organic agriculture uses energy much more efficiently and greatly reduces carbon dioxide (CO_2) emissions compared with conventional agriculture, both with respect to direct energy consumption in fuel and oil and indirect consumption in synthetic fertilizers and pesticides.

Sustainable agriculture restores soil organic matter content, increasing carbon sequestration below ground, thereby recovering an important carbon sink. Organic systems have shown significant ability to absorb and retain carbon, raising the possibility that sustainable agriculture practices can help reduce the impact of global warming.

Organic agriculture is likely to emit less nitrous oxide (N_2O), another important greenhouse gas and a cause of stratospheric ozone depletion as well.

8. Efficient and profitable production

Any yield reduction in organic agriculture is more than offset by ecological and efficiency gains. Research has shown that the organic approach can be commercially viable in the long-term, producing more food per unit of energy or resources.

Data show that smaller farms produce far more per unit area than the larger farms characteristic of conventional farming. Though the yield per unit area of one crop may be lower on a small farm than on a large monoculture, the total output per unit area, often composed of over a dozen crops and various animal products, can be far higher.

Production costs for organic farming are often lower than for conventional farming, bringing equivalent or higher net returns even without organic price premiums. When price premiums are factored in, organic systems are almost always more profitable.

9. Improved food security and benefits to local communities
A review of sustainable agriculture projects in developing countries showed that average food production per household increased by 1.71 tons per year (up 73%) for 4.42 million farmers on 3.58 million hectares, bringing food security and health benefits.

Increasing agricultural productivity has been shown to also increase food supplies and raise incomes, thereby reducing poverty, increasing access to food, reducing malnutrition and improving health and livelihoods.

Sustainable agricultural approaches draw extensively on traditional and indigenous knowledge, and place emphasis on the farmers' experience and innovation. This thereby utilizes appropriate, low-cost and readily available local resources as well as improves farmers' status and autonomy, enhancing social and cultural relations within local communities.

Local means of sale and distribution can generate more money for the local economy. For every £1 spent at an organic box scheme from Cusgarne Organics (UK), £2.59 is generated for the local economy; but for every £1 spent at a supermarket, only £1.40 is generated for the local economy.

10. Better food quality for health
Organic food is safer, as organic farming prohibits routine pesticide and herbicide use, so harmful chemical residues are rarely found.

Organic production also bans the use of artificial food additives such as hydrogenated fats, phosphoric acid, aspartame and monosodium glutamate, which have been linked to health problems as diverse as heart disease, osteoporosis, migraines and hyperactivity.

Studies have shown that, on average, organic food has higher vitamin C, higher mineral levels and higher plant phenolics—plant compounds that can fight cancer and heart disease, and combat age-related neurological dysfunctions—and significantly less nitrates, a toxic compound.

Sustainable agricultural practices have proven beneficial in all aspects relevant to health and the environment. In addition, they bring food security and social and cultural well-being to local communities everywhere. There is an urgent need for a comprehensive global shift to all forms of sustainable agriculture.

Part 1: No Future for GM Crops

1

Why Not GM Crops?

GM Crops Are Neither Needed Nor Wanted

There is no longer any doubt that genetically modified (GM) crops are not needed to feed the world, and that hunger is caused by poverty and inequality, not by inadequate production of food. According to estimates by the Food and Agriculture Organization of the United Nations (FAO), there is enough food produced to feed everyone *using only conventional crops*, and that will remain the case for at least 25 years and probably far into the future [2].

Furthermore, as Altieri and Rosset have argued, even if hunger is due to a gap between food production and human population growth, current GM crops are not designed to increase yields, nor for growth by the poor, small farmers, so they are unlikely to benefit from them [3]. Because the true root cause of hunger is inequality, any method of boosting food production that deepens inequality is bound to fail to reduce hunger [4]. A recent report by ActionAid concludes that "The widespread adoption of GM crops seems likely to exacerbate the underlying cause of food insecurity, leading to more hungry people, not fewer" [5].

More importantly, GM crops are not wanted, and for good reasons. GM crops have failed to deliver the promised benefits, they are causing escalating problems on the farm, and evidence of the worst hazards has accumulated despite the notable lack of research on safety. At the same time, extensive evidence has emerged on the success of sustainable approaches to agriculture, which makes clear what the rational choice for any nation ought to be.

The world market for GM crops has been shrinking simultaneously with sharply increasing yields since the first GM crop, the Flavr Savr™ tomato, was planted in the United States (US) in 1994—a product soon withdrawn as a commercial disaster. During the seven-year period from 1996 to 2002, the global acreage of GM crops increased from 1.7 million hectares to 58.7 million hectares. But only

3

four countries accounted for 99% of the global GM-crop acreage in 2002. The US grew 39.0 million hectares, (66% of the global total), Argentina 13.5 million hectares, Canada 3.5 million hectares and China 2.1 million hectares [6].

Worldwide resistance to GM crops reached a climax last year when Zambia refused GM maize (corn) in food aid despite the threat of famine. Zambia has since reaffirmed its decision after a high-level delegation was invited to visit several countries, including the US and the United Kingdom (UK). As we were drafting this report, a hunger strike was in progress in the Philippines, protesting the commercial approval of Monsanto's Bt maize.

Citizen juries and other participatory democracy and social inclusion processes have been used in India, Zimbabwe and Brazil to allow small farmers and marginalized rural communities to assess the risks and desirability of GM crops on their own terms and according to their own criteria and notions of well-being.

The results show that when and where these events have been facilitated in a trustworthy, credible and unbiased manner, small farmers and indigenous peoples have rejected GM crops on the grounds that they do not need them, and that the GM technology is unproven and does not meet their needs [7, 8].

The agricultural sector led the dramatic decline of the biotech industry before the industry peaked in 2000 on the back of the human genome project. The Institute of Science in Society (ISIS) has summarized the evidence in a special briefing to the UK Prime Minister's Strategy Unit on GM crops, submitted in response to its public consultation on the economic potential of GM crops [9]. Since then, things have gotten worse for the entire industry [10].

A report released in April 2003 by Innovest Strategic Value Advisors [11] gave Monsanto the lowest possible rating with the message that agricultural biotechnology is a high-risk industry not worth investing in unless it changes its focus away from GE (genetic engineering, synonymous with GM). The report states:

"Money flowing from GE companies to politicians as well as the frequency with which GE company employees take jobs with US regulatory agencies (and vice versa) creates large bias potential and reduces the ability of investors to rely on safety claims made by the US Government. It also helps to clarify why the US Government has not taken a precautionary approach to GE and continues to suppress GE labeling in the face of overwhelming public support for it. With Enron and other financial disasters, the financial community apparently bought into company stories without looking much below the surface. . . ."

"Monsanto could be another disaster waiting to happen for investors," the report concludes.

GM Crops Failed to Deliver the Benefits

GM crops have simply not delivered the promised benefits. That is the consistent finding of independent research and on-farm surveys, reviewed by agronomist Charles Benbrook in the US since 1999 [12, 13], and other studies have borne this out [14].

Thousands of controlled trials of GM soya gave significantly decreased yields of between 5 to 10%, and in some locations as much as 12 to 20% compared with non-GM soya. Similar reductions in yield have been reported in Britain for GM winter oilseed rape (canola) and sugar beet in field trials.

GM crops have not resulted in significant reductions in herbicide and insecticide/pesticide use. Roundup Ready™ (RR) soya required 2 to 5 times more herbicide (measured in pounds applied per acre) than other weed management systems. Similarly, US Department of Agriculture (USDA) data suggest that in 2000 the average acre of RR maize was treated with 30% more herbicide than the average acre of non-GM maize.

Analysis of four years of official USDA data on insecticide use shows a pretty clear picture [13]. While Bt cotton has reduced insecticide use in several states, Bt corn (maize) has had little, if any, impacts on corn insecticide use. USDA data show that corn insecticide applications directly targeting the European corn borer increased from about 4% of acres treated in 1995 to about 5% in 2000.

The greater cost of GM seeds, the increased herbicide/pesticide use, yield drag, royalties on seed and reduced markets, all add up to lost income for farmers. The first farm-level economic analysis of Bt maize in the US revealed that between 1996 and 2001 the net loss to farmers was $92 million or about $1.31 per acre.

A UK Soil Association report [15] released in September 2002, estimated that GM crops have cost the United States $12 billion in farm subsidies, lost sales and product recalls due to transgenic contamination. It summed up as follows:

"The evidence we set out suggests that . . . virtually every benefit claimed for GM crops has not occurred. Instead, farmers are reporting lower yields, continuing dependency on herbicides and pesticides, loss of access to markets and, critically, reduced profitability leaving food production even more vulnerable to the interests of the biotechnology companies and in need of subsidies."

These studies have not taken into account crop failures elsewhere in the world, the most serious occurring in India last year [16]. Massive failures of GM cotton, up to 100%, were reported in several Indian states, including failure to germinate, root-rot and attacks by the American bollworm, for which the Bt cotton was supposed to be resistant.

2

Escalating Problems on the Farm

Transgenic Instability

The massive failures of GM cotton in India, and of other GM crops elsewhere, are most likely due to the fact that GM crops are overwhelmingly unstable, a problem first highlighted in a 1994 review by Finnegan and McElroy [17]:

"While there are some examples of plants which show stable expression of a transgene these may prove to be the exceptions to the rule. In an informal survey of over 30 companies involved in the commercialization of transgenic crop plants . . . almost all of the respondents indicated that they had observed some level of transgene inaction. Many respondents indicated that most cases of transgene inactivation never reach the literature."

There is, nevertheless, substantial scientific literature on transgenic instability [18, 19]. Whenever the appropriate molecular tools have been applied to investigate the problem, instability is invariably found, and that is so even in cases where transgenic *stability* has been claimed. In one publication [20], which stated in the abstract that "transgene expression was stable in lines of all the rice genotypes," the data presented actually showed that, *at most, 7 out of 40 (18%) of the lines may be stable to the R3 generation* [21]. This paper, like many others, also misused the failure to deviate significantly from arbitrarily set "Mendelian ratios" as a sign of Mendelian inheritance, or genetic stability. This is such an elementary mistake in statistics and genetics that students could fail an exam for making it.

There are two major causes of transgenic instability. The first has to do with the defence mechanisms protecting the integrity of the organism that "silence" or inactivate foreign genes integrated into the genome, so that they are no longer expressed. Gene silencing was first discovered in connection with integrated transgenes in the early 1990s, and is now known to be part of the organism's defence against viral infections.

The second major cause of instability has to do with the *structural* instability of the transgenic constructs themselves, their tendency to fragment, to break along weak artificial joints and to recombine incorrectly, often with other DNA that happens to be around. That is perhaps more serious from the safety point of view, as it enhances horizontal gene transfer and recombination (see later).

Yet another source of instability has been more recently discovered [18]. There appear to be certain "receptive hotspots" for transgenic integration in both the plant and the human genomes. These receptive hotspots may also be "recombination hotspots," prone to breaking and rejoining. That, too, would make inserted transgenes more likely to come loose again, to recombine, or to invade other genomes.

Investigations also show that transgene instability may arise in later generations, and is not necessarily "selected out" during early generations of growth. This can result in poor and inconsistent performances of the GM crops in the field, a problem likely to be underreported by farmers who settle for compensation with a gagging clause.

Stop the Press

A newly published report (Makarevitch I., S. D. Svitashev, and D. A. Somers. Complete sequence analysis of transgene loci from plants transformed via microprojectile bombardment. *Plant Molecular Biology*, 2003, 52, 421–32) reveals that the problem associated with the uncontrollable and unpredictable integration of transgenes is even worse than it seems, and GE can in no way be equated with conventional breeding or mutagenesis.

The authors point out that the majority of transgenic lines produced by microprojectile bombardment have "complex transgene loci composed of multiple copies of whole, truncated, and rearranged delivered DNAs frequently organized as direct or inverted repeats that are interspersed with variable-sized genomic DNA fragments" and that the delivered DNA is integrated into plant genomes primarily through "illegitimate recombination (IR) associated with double-strand break (DSB) repair, a process also involved in integration of T-DNA into yeast and plant genomes."

They also note that "The hallmarks of IR in transgene loci produced via direct DNA delivery include scrambling of transgene sequences through recombination of both large and small noncontiguous fragments of the delivered DNA, frequent incorporation of genomic DNA sequences into the transgene loci and rearrangement in the genomic DNA flanking the transgene locus."

The target sites frequently cannot be fully characterized because of translocations and deletions in the adjacent genomic DNA. That means it is not even possible to tell where in the genome the transgene has integrated, even if the entire sequence of the host genome is known.

The researchers have completely sequenced a few transgene loci in transgenic oat that appear to be "simple," and hence may be closer to having the expected gene order and normal flanking genome sequences.

Unfortunately, all three "simple" loci possess regions of small scrambled fragments of delivered and genomic DNA. All loci also exhibited either scrambled filler DNA (unknown origin) flanking the transgene DNA or evidence of deletion of the target site DNA.

One of the transgenic lines studied was previously characterized and shown to have a single major locus estimated to be about 15 kb in length. However, the T1 progeny analyzed by southern blot with longer exposure times and more genomic DNA gave two additional minor transgene loci.

Southern analysis showed that the genomic DNA flanking both sides of one of the loci was highly repetitive. Aligning the product of Polymerase Chain Reaction (PCR—a method for amplifying specific DNA sequences) of transgene locus with wild type showed that 845 bp of genomic DNA were deleted from the wild-type genome during transgene integration and that pieces of genomic DNA of unknown origin were integrated into the locus as filler DNA on both sides of the transgene DNA.

The target sites of the other two loci could not be identified on account of extensive scrambling of the genomic DNA. The authors also point out, "it is now accepted that transgene locus number estimations based on phenotypic segregation ratios are inaccurate due to perturbations of transgene expression via transgene silencing or rearrangements of transgene loci." Depending on the probe used, small, nonfunctional loci are simply not detected.

Integration sites are worse than random. There is evidence that transgene DNA often gets into gene-rich regions and regions prone to double-stranded breaks. The former increases the potential of activating/inactivating genes, and the latter increases the structural instability of transgenes and transgenic lines.

Volunteers and Weeds

Triple herbicide-tolerant oilseed rape volunteers were first discovered in 1998 in Alberta, Canada, just two years after single herbicide-tolerant GM crops were planted [22]. A year later, these multiple herbicide-tolerant volunteers were found in 11 other fields [23]. The US only started growing herbicide-tolerant GM oilseed rape in 2001. Research at Idaho University reported that similar multiple gene-stacking had occurred in experimental plots over two years and, during the same period, weeds with two herbicide-tolerance traits were also found.

Many other problems with weeds have been identified since (summarized in ref. 24). Glyphosate-resistant marestail infested over 200,000 acres of cotton in western Tennessee (USA) in 2002, or 36% of all cotton acreage in the state, and some 200,000 acres of soya beans were also affected. The problem with herbicide-tolerant volunteers and weeds is such that companies have been recommending spraying with additional herbicides. US agricultural experts reveal that between 75% and 90% of GM maize growers are using a product called Liberty ATZ™—a mixture of Aventis's weed killer, glufosinate ammonium, and Atrazine, the traditional herbicide used on maize crops that has been a problem pesticide for decades [25]. Atrazine is on Europe's Red List and Priority List for hormone-disrupting effects in animals. Glufosinate itself is far from benign (see later).

Bt crops are also experiencing problems from resistance that is likely to develop in target pests (see below). A new patent application from Monsanto is based on using two insecticides with their Bt crops, on the grounds that Bt crops could produce resistant strains of insect pests and "numerous problems remain . . . under actual field conditions."

Recent research shows that transgenes from Bt sunflower crossing into wild relatives made the latter hardier and more prolific, with the potential of becoming superweeds [26].

Bt Resistance

Bt crops are genetically engineered to produce insecticidal proteins derived from genes of the bacterium *Bacillus thuringiensis* (Bt). The likelihood of target pests of Bt crops developing resistance to Bt toxins rapidly is so great and real that, in the US, resistance management strategies are adopted, involving planting "refugia" of non-Bt crops and developing Bt crops with high levels of expression, or multiple toxins, in the same crop.

Unfortunately, pests have developed resistance to multiple toxins, or cross-resistances to different toxins [27], and recent research reveals that resistant strains are even able to obtain additional nutritional value from the toxin, thus possibly making them more serious pests than before.

Extensive Transgenic Contamination

In November 2001, Berkeley plant geneticists Ignacio Chapela and David Quist published a report in *Nature* [28] presenting evidence that maize landraces*, growing in remote regions in Mexico, were contaminated with transgenes, despite the fact that an official moratorium on growing GM maize has been imposed in the country.

This sparked off a concerted attack by pro-biotech scientists, allegedly orchestrated by Monsanto [29]. *Nature* withdrew support for that paper in February 2002, an act unprecedented in the history of scientific publication for a paper that was neither wrong nor challenged on its major conclusion. Subsequent research by Mexican scientists confirmed the finding, showing that the contamination was much more extensive than previously suspected [30]. Ninety-five percent of the sites sampled were contaminated, with degrees of contamination varying from 1 to 35% (averaging 10 to 15%). The companies involved have refused to provide molecular information or probes for research, which would sort out which are the liable parties for the damages caused. *Nature* refused to publish these confirmatory results.

Indeed, one main factor considered by the Innovest report (see above) that would damn Monsanto is the substantial investor losses that could arise from unintended transgenic contamination. *Contamination is inevitable, the report states, and could bankrupt Monsanto and other biotech companies, leaving the rest of society to deal with the problem.*

According to Ignacio Chapela, who finds himself caught up in the ensuing controversy with his University tenure still hanging in the balance, transgenic contamination in Mexico is still growing.

The extent of contamination of non-GM seeds is alarming. A spokesperson from Dow Agroscience was reported as saying that "the whole seed system is contaminated" in Canada [31]. Dr. Lyle Friesen of the University of Manitoba tested 33 samples representing

27 pedigreed canola (oilseed rape) seed stocks and found 32 were contaminated [32].

Tests on pollen flow found that wheat pollen will stay airborne for one hour at the minimum, which means it could be carried huge distances depending on the wind speed. Canola pollen is even lighter and can remain airborne for 3 to 6 hours. A 35 mile/hour wind is not atypical, which "makes a real mockery of a separation distance of tens or even hundreds of meters," said Percy Schmeiser, celebrated Canadian farmer who was ordered by the Canadian court to pay "damages" to Monsanto, despite his claim that his neighbor's GM crop had contaminated his fields. Schmeiser lost his appeal in the Federal Court, but has just won his right to be heard in the Supreme Court of Canada.

Organic farmers in Saskatchewan have also started legal proceedings against Monsanto and Aventis for contaminating their crops and ruining their organic status.

The European Commission ordered the study on the coexistence of GM and non-GM crops in May 2000 from the Institute for Prospective Technological Studies of the EU Joint Research Centre. The study was completed and delivered to the European Commission in January 2002 with the recommendation that it *not* be made public. The suppressed study, leaked to Greenpeace [33], confirmed what we already know: *coexistence of GM farming and non-GM, or organic farming, would be impossible in many cases.* Even in cases where it is technically feasible, it would require costly measures to avoid contamination and increase production costs for all farmers, especially small farmers.

Transgenic contamination is not limited to cross-pollination. New research shows that transgenic pollen, wind-blown and deposited elsewhere, or that has fallen directly to the ground, is a major source of transgenic contamination [34]. Such transgenic DNA was even found in fields where GM crops have never been grown, and soil samples contaminated with pollen were demonstrated to transfer transgenic DNA to soil bacteria (see later).

Why is contamination such a big issue? The immediate answer is that consumers are not accepting it. The more important reason is that there are outstanding safety concerns.

Part 2: GM Crops Are Not Safe

3

Science and Precaution

Precaution, Common Sense and Science

We are told there is no scientific evidence that GM is harmful. But is it safe? That is the question we should ask. Where something can cause serious irreversible harm, it is right and proper for scientists to demand evidence demonstrating that GM is safe *beyond reasonable doubt*. That is usually dignified as "the precautionary principle," but for scientists and for the public, it is just common sense [35–37].

Scientific evidence is no different from ordinary evidence and should be understood and judged in the same way. Evidence from different sources and of different kinds has to be weighed and combined to guide policy decisions and actions. That's good science as well as good sense.

Genetic engineering involves recombining (i.e., joining together in new combinations) DNA from different sources and inserting them into the genomes of organisms to make "genetically modified organisms," or "GMOs" [38].

GMOs are unnatural, not just because they have been produced in the laboratory, but because many of them can *only* be made in the laboratory, quite unlike what nature has produced in the course of billions of years of evolution.

Thus, it is possible to introduce new genes and gene products—many from bacteria, viruses and other species, or even genes made entirely in the laboratory—into crops, including food crops. We have never eaten these new genes and gene products, nor have they ever been part of our food chain.

The artificial constructs are introduced into cells by invasive methods that result in random integration into the genome, giving rise to unpredictable, random effects, including gross abnormalities in both animals and plants, and unexpected toxins and allergens in food crops. In other words, there is no possibility for quality control.

This problem is compounded by the overwhelming instability of transgenic lines, which makes risk assessment virtually impossible.

Anti-precautionary Risk Assessment

Many of the problems would have been identified if regulators had taken risk assessment seriously. But as pointed out by Ho and Steinbrecher [39], there were fatal flaws in the procedure of food safety assessment from the start, as laid down in the Joint FAO/WHO Biotechnology and Food Safety Report resulting from an Expert Consultation in Rome, September 30 to October 4, 1996, which has served as the main model ever since.

That report was criticized for:

- Making contentious claims for the benefits of the technology.
- Failing to assume responsibility for or to address major aspects of food safety, such as the use of food crops for producing pharmaceuticals and industrial chemicals, as well as issues of labeling and monitoring.
- Restricting the scope of safety considerations to exclude known hazards, such as the toxicity of broad-spectrum herbicides.
- Claiming erroneously that genetic engineering does not differ from conventional breeding.
- Using a "principle of substantial equivalence" for risk assessment that is both arbitrary and unscientific.
- Failing to address long-term impacts on health and food security.
- Ignoring existing scientific findings on identifiable hazards, especially those resulting from the horizontal transfer and recombination of transgenic DNA.

All that makes for an *anti*-precautionary "safety assessment" that is designed to expedite product approval at the expense of safety considerations.

The Principle of "Substantial Equivalence" Is a Sham in Terms of Risk Assessment

The biggest faults are in the principle of "substantial equivalence" that is supposed to serve as the backbone of risk assessment. The report stated,

"Substantial equivalence embodies the concept that, if a new food or food component is found to be substantially equivalent to an existing food or food component, it can be treated in the same manner with respect to safety (i.e., the food or food component can be concluded to be as safe as the conventional food or food component)."

As can be seen, the principle is vague and ill-defined. But what follows makes clear that it is intended to be as flexible, malleable and open to interpretation as possible.

"Establishment of substantial equivalence is not a safety assessment in itself, but a dynamic, analytical exercise in the assessment of the safety of a new food relative to an existing food. The comparison may be a simple task or be very lengthy depending upon the amount of available knowledge and the nature of the food or food component under consideration. The reference characteristics for substantial equivalence comparisons need to be flexible and will change over time in accordance with the changing needs of processors and consumers and with experience."

In other words, there would be neither required nor specified tests for establishing substantial equivalence (SE). Companies would be free to compare whatever is the most expeditious for claiming SE, and to carry out the least discriminating tests that would conceal any substantial difference.

In practice, the principle of SE has allowed the companies to:

- Do the least discriminating tests, such as crude compositions of proteins, carbohydrates, fats, amino acids and selected metabolites.
- Avoid detailed molecular characterization of the transgenic insert to establish genetic stability, gene expression profiles, metabolic profiles, etc., that would have revealed unintended effects.
- Claim that the transgenic line is substantially equivalent to the nontransgenic line except for the transgene product, and to carry out risk assessment solely on the transgene product, thereby, again, ignoring any and all unintended changes.
- Avoid comparing the transgenic line to its nontransgenic "parent" grown under the same range of environmental conditions.
- Compare the transgenic line to any variety within the species, and even to an abstract entity made up of the composite of selected characteristics from all varieties within the species,

so that the transgenic line could have the worst features of every variety and still be considered SE.

• Compare different components of a transgenic line with different species, as in the case of a transgenic canola engineered to produce lauric acid. But "other fatty acids components are Generally Recognized as Safe (GRAS) when evaluated individually because they are present at similar levels in other commonly consumed oils."

No wonder the report could go on to state, "Up to the present time, and probably for the near future, there have been few, if any, examples of foods or food components produced using genetic modification which could be considered to be not substantially equivalent to existing foods or food components."

Transgenic instability makes regulation based on this principle of SE even more ridiculous. A paper presented a year earlier at a WHO workshop [40] stated, "The main difficulty associated with the biosafety assessment of transgenic crops is the unpredictable nature of transformation. The unpredictability raises the concern that transgenic plants will behave in an inconsistent manner when grown commercially." Consequently, transgenic potatoes, which on field trials "showed marked deformities in shoot morphology and poor tuber yield involving a low number of small, malformed tubers" nonetheless gave "virtually no changes in tuber quality" under the tests applied, and was therefore passed as "substantially equivalent."

Contrary to what has been widely claimed, therefore, GM foods have never passed any required tests that could have established they are safe. The Food and Drug Administration (FDA) in the US had decided in 1992 that genetic engineering was just an extension of conventional breeding and therefore safety assessments were unnecessary. Although the first transgenic crop, Flavr Savr™ tomato, went through a nominal safety assessment (which it failed, see later), all subsequent crops went through a voluntary consultation procedure.

Belinda Martineau, the scientist who conducted the safety studies on Flavr Savr™ tomato at the company Calgene, has published a book [41] in which she stated that "Calgene's tomato should not serve as a safety standard for this new industry. No single genetically engineered product should." She strongly decries the lack of data on health and environmental impacts of transgenic crops. "And simply proclaiming that 'these foods are safe and there is no scientific evidence to the contrary' is not the same as saying 'extensive tests have been conducted and here are the results.'"

The US National Academy of Sciences (NAS) released a report in February 2002 criticizing the USDA for inadequately protecting the environment from the risks of GM plants [42]. It said that the USDA review processes lack scientific justification and are not applied uniformly; the assessment of environmental risks, particularly from plants genetically engineered to be insect resistant, was "generally superficial"; and the process "hampers external review and transparency" by keeping environmental assessments confidential as trade secrets. The report calls on the USDA to make its review process "significantly more transparent and rigorous," to seek evaluation of its findings from outside scientific experts and to solicit greater input from the public.

There are, indeed, very few independent studies dedicated to the safety of GM crops to health and the environment. Nevertheless, sufficient evidence has accumulated to indicate that GM crops are not safe.

We are definitely well into the early warning period at which common sense, or the application of the precautionary principle, can still avert and ameliorate the disasters that are likely to occur in the longer term [43].

4

Safety Tests on GM Foods

Paucity of Published Data

There is a distinct scarcity of published data relevant to the safety of GM foods. Not only that, the scientific quality of what has been published is, in most instances, not up to the usually expected standards of good science.

In responding to the Scottish Parliament's recent investigation into the health impacts of GM crops [44], Stanley Ewen, histopathologist at Grampian University Hospital Trust, and leader of the Colorectal Cancer Screening Pilot in Grampian Region, summed up the situation,

"It is unfortunate that very few animal trials of GM human food are available in the public domain in scientific literature. It follows that GM foods have not been shown to be without risk and, indeed, the available scientific experimental results demonstrate cause for concern."

Two reports prior to 1999 revealed harmful effects on animals fed GM foods. The first was a report submitted to the US FDA on Flavr Savr™ GM tomatoes fed to rats. Several of the rats developed erosions (early ulcers) of the lining of the stomach similar to those seen in the stomach of older humans on aspirin or similar medication. In humans, substantial life-threatening hemorrhage may occur from these early ulcers.

The second paper, published in a peer-reviewed journal, was on feeding raw GM potatoes to month-old male mice. The results revealed proliferative growth in the lower small intestine [45].

The Study by Pusztai and Coworkers

No substantive studies on the health impacts of GM food had been carried out until what was the Scottish Office of Agriculture, Environment and Fisheries Department (SOAEFD) funded the project headed by Arpad Pusztai at the Rowett Institute to undertake a major investigation into the possible environmental and health hazards of GM potatoes that had been transformed by British scientists using a gene taken from snowdrop bulbs [46].

The studies revealed that the two transgenic lines of GM potatoes, which originated from the same transformation experiment, and were both resistant to aphid pests, were *not* substantially equivalent in composition to parent-line potatoes, nor to each other. The crude, poorly defined and unscientific concept of "substantial equivalence" that regulators rely on in risk assessment has been criticized from its conception (see above). It has certainly outlived its usefulness.

More importantly, the results showed that diets containing GM potatoes had, in some instances, interfered with the growth of the young rats and the development of some of their vital organs, inducing changes in gut structure and function, and reducing their immune responsiveness to injurious antigens. In contrast, the animals fed on diets containing the parent, non-GM potatoes, or these potatoes supplemented with the gene product, had no such effects. Some of the results have been published since [47–51]. The latest paper [51] is a comprehensive review on safety tests involving GM foods, including the unpublished experiments on GM tomatoes submitted to the FDA, described earlier.

The findings of Pusztai and colleagues have been attacked by many within the scientific establishment, but never disproved by repeating the work and publishing the results in peer-reviewed journals. They have clearly demonstrated that it is possible to perform toxicological studies, and that the safety of GM foodstuffs must be established in short- and long-term feeding, metabolic and immune-response studies with *young* animals, as these are most vulnerable and the most likely to respond to, and display, any nutritional and metabolic stresses affecting development—a view shared by other scientists.

Multivariate statistical analysis of the results carried out independently by Scottish Agricultural Statistics Service suggested that the major potentially harmful effects of the GM potatoes were only in part caused by the presence of the snowdrop lectin transgene, and that the method of genetic transformation, and/or the disturbances in the potato genome, also made major contributions to the changes observed.

Ewen and Pusztai's paper, published in *The Lancet* [48], aroused much controversy, and it seems that attempts to discredit Pusztai by members of the Royal Society continue to the present day.

Ewen and Pusztai measured the part of the small bowel lining that produces new cells and found that the length of the new cell compartment had increased significantly in GM-fed rats, but not in control rats fed non-GM potatoes. The increased production of cells had to be due to a growth-factor effect induced by the genetic modification within the potatoes. (Growth factors are proteins that promote cell growth and multiplication that, if uncontrolled, result in cancer.) Similar effects were observed in the stomach lining [51].

Statistical analysis further revealed that the growth-factor effect was not due to the expressed transgenic protein, the snowdrop lectin, but was the effect of the gene construct inserted into the DNA of the potato genome. In other words, non-GM potatoes spiked with snowdrop lectin simply did not have the same effect.

The construct includes not only the new gene, but also marker genes and a powerful promoter from the cauliflower mosaic virus (CaMV), which is at the center of a major debate concerning its safety (see later).

Ewen [44] pointed out that although the whole and intact virus appears to be harmless, as we have been eating cauliflower-type vegetables for millennia, "the use of the separate infectious part of the virus has not been tested in animals."

Further possible undesirable effects may involve the human liver's response to hepatitis virus, as the cauliflower mosaic virus and hepatitis B virus belong to the same family of pararetroviruses, with closely similar genomes and a distinctive life cycle.

That and other potential hazards of the CaMV promoter will be dealt with in more detail later.

5

Transgene Hazards

Bt Toxins

The most obvious question on safety is with regard to the transgene and its product introduced into GM crops, as they are new to the ecosystem and to the food chain of animals and human beings. The Bt toxins from *Bacillus thuringiensis*, incorporated into food and nonfood crops, account for about 25% of all GM crops currently grown worldwide. It was found to be harmful to mice, butterflies and lacewings up the food chain [27]. Bt toxins also act against insects in the Order of Coleoptera (beetles, weevils and styloplids), which contains some 28,600 species, far more than any other Order. Bt plants exude the toxin through the roots into the soil, with potentially large impacts on soil ecology and fertility.

Bt toxins may be actual and potential allergens for human beings. Some field workers exposed to Bt spray experienced allergic skin sensitization and produced IgE and IgG antibodies. A team of scientists has cautioned against releasing Bt crops for human use. They demonstrated that recombinant Cry1Ac protoxin from Bt is a potent systemic and mucosal immunogen, as potent as cholera toxin [52].

A Bt strain that caused severe human necrosis (tissue death) killed mice within 8 hours from clinical toxic-shock syndrome [53]. Both Bt protein and Bt potatoes harmed mice in feeding experiments, damaging their ileum (part of the small intestine) [45]. The mice showed abnormal mitochondria, with signs of degeneration and disrupted microvilli (microscopic projections on the cell surface) at the surface lining the gut.

Because Bt or *Bacillus thuringiensis* and *Bacillus anthracis* (anthrax species used in biological weapons) are closely related to each other and to a third bacterium, *Bacillus cereus*, a common soil bacterium that causes food poisoning, they can readily exchange plasmids (circular DNA molecules containing genetic origins of replication that allow replication independent of the chromosome) carrying toxin genes [54]. If *B. anthracis* picked up Bt genes from Bt crops by horizontal gene transfer (see later), new strains of *B. anthracis* with unpredictable properties could arise.

"Pharm" crops

Other hazardous genes and bacterial and viral sequences are incorporated into our food and nonfood crops as vaccines and pharmaceuticals in "next generation" GM crops [55–62]. These pharm crops include those expressing cytokines, known to suppress the immune system, induce sickness and central nervous system toxicity, as well as interferon alpha, which is reported to cause dementia, neurotoxicity and mood and cognitive side effects. Some contain viral sequences such as the "spike" protein gene of the pig corona virus, in the same family as the SARS virus linked to the current global epidemic [63, 64].

The glycoprotein gene *gp120* of the AIDS virus HIV-1, incorporated into GM maize as a "cheap, edible oral vaccine," is yet another biological time-bomb. There is a lot of evidence that this gene can interfere with the immune system, as it has homology to the antigen-binding variable regions of the immunoglobulins, and has recombination sites similar to those of the immunoglobulins. Furthermore, these recombination sites are also similar to the recombination sites present in many viruses and bacteria, with which the *gp120* can recombine to generate deadly pathogens [65–68].

Bacterial and viral DNA

A previously neglected source of hazard in GM crops—though not in gene therapy where it is recognized as something to avoid—is the DNA from bacteria and their viruses, which have a high frequency of the CpG dinucleotide [24]. These CpG motifs are immunogenic and can cause inflammation, septic arthritis and promotion of B cell lymphoma and autoimmune disease [69–73]. Still, many genes introduced into GMOs are from bacteria and their viruses, and these pose other risks as well (see below).

6

Terminator Crops
Spread Male Sterility

"Suicide" Genes for Sterility

In the interest of avoiding tedious semantic arguments, "terminator crops" here refer to any transgenic crop engineered with a "suicide" gene for male, female or seed sterility, for the purpose of preventing farmers from saving and replanting seeds, or protecting patented traits.

The public first became aware of terminator technology in patents jointly owned by the USDA and Delta and Pine Land Company. That engendered massive protests worldwide, and Monsanto, which acquired the Delta and Pine Land patent rights, backed down from developing the terminator crops *described in that particular patent*. However, as Ho and Cummins were to learn, there are many ways to engineer sterility, each the subject of a separate patent.

It turned out that terminator crops have been field tested in Europe, Canada and the US since the early 1990s, and several were already commercially released in North America [74]. The GM oilseed rape, both spring and winter varieties, which form the main part of the Farm Scale Evaluations in the UK, are engineered to be male sterile.

GM Oilseed Rapes Are Terminator Crops

The male sterility system in these GM oilseed rapes consists of three lines.

The *male-sterile line* is maintained in a "hemizygous" state (i.e., with only one copy of the "suicide" gene, *barnase*, joined to a glufosinate-tolerant gene.) The *barnase* gene is driven from a promoter (gene switch) that's active only in the anther or male part of the flower. The expression of the *barnase* gene in the anther gives rise to the protein barnase, an RNAse (enzyme that breaks down RNA), which is a potent cell poison. The cell dies and stops anther development, so no pollen is produced. This male-sterile line is perpetrated in the hemizygous state by crossing to a non-GM variety and using glufosinate ammonium to kill off half the plants in the offspring generation that do not have a copy of the *H-barnase* transgene joined to it.

The *male-restorer line* is homozygous (with two copies) for the "sterility-restorer" gene, *barstar*, also joined to the glufosinate-tolerant gene. The *barstar* gene, too, is placed under the control of the special promoter that's active in the anther. Its expression gives the barstar protein that's a specific inhibitor of barnase, thereby neutralizing the latter's activity.

Crossing the male-sterile line to the male-restorer line produces an *F1 hybrid*, in which the barnase is neutralized by barstar, thus restoring anther development to produce pollen.

It can be shown that the F1 hybrid actually spreads both the herbicide-tolerance gene and the suicide gene for male sterility in its pollen, with potentially devastating impacts on both agricultural and natural biodiversity. It makes a mockery of the UK and US governments' promotion of these plants as a way to "contain" or "prevent" the spread of transgenes. The real purpose of this kind of terminator engineering is to protect corporate patents.

7

Herbicide Hazards

Herbicide Profits

More than 75% of all GM crops currently grown worldwide are engineered to be tolerant to broad-spectrum herbicides manufactured by the same companies that make most of their profits from sales of the herbicides. These broad-spectrum herbicides not only kill plants indiscriminately, they are also harmful to practically all species of animal wildlife and to human beings.

Glufosinate Ammonium

Glufosinate ammonium, or phosphinothricin, is linked to neurological, respiratory, gastrointestinal and hematological toxicities as well as birth defects in humans and mammals [75]. It is toxic to butterflies and a number of beneficial insects, also to the larvae of clams and oysters, *Daphnia* and some freshwater fish, especially the rainbow trout. It inhibits beneficial soil bacteria and fungi that fix nitrogen.

The loss of insects and plants would have knock-on effects on birds and small animal life.

In addition, some plant pathogens were found to be highly resistant to glufosinate while organisms antagonistic to those pathogens were seriously and adversely affected. This could have catastrophic impacts on agriculture.

The glufosinate-tolerant plants contain the *pat* (phosphinothricin acetyl transferase) gene, which inactivates phosphinothricin by adding an acetyl group to it to make acetylphosphinothricin. The latter accumulates in the GM plant and is a completely new metabolite in the crop, as well as for the entire food chain leading up to human beings, the risks of which have not been considered.

Data supplied by AgrEvo, which became Aventis and now Bayer CropScience, show that microorganisms in the gut of warm-blooded animals can remove the acetyl group and regenerate the toxic herbicide. Phosphinothricin inhibits the enzyme glutamine synthetase, which converts the essential amino acid, glutamic acid, to glutamine. The net result of the action of glufosinate is that ammonia and glutamate accumulate at the expense of glutamine. It is the accumulation of ammonia that is the lethal action in plants.

In mammals, the consequences of inhibition of glutamine synthetase are more associated with the increased levels of glutamate, and decreased levels of glutamine. Circulating ammonia is removed in the liver by the urea cycle. However, the brain is highly sensitive to the toxic effects of ammonia, and the removal of excess ammonia depends on its incorporation into glutamine. Glutamate is a major neurotransmitter, and such a large disturbance to its metabolism is bound to impact health.

These known effects are sufficient to halt all field trials of GM crops immediately, until critical questions about the metabolism, storage and reconversion of the N-acetylphosphinothricin have been fully answered for *all pat* gene-containing products.

Glyphosate

The other major herbicide used in conjunction with GM crops, glyphosate, is no better [76].

Glyphosate kills plants by inhibiting the enzyme 5-enolpyruvyl-shikimate-3-phosphate synthetase (EPSPS), critical for the biosynthesis of aromatic amino acids such as phenylalanine, tyrosine and tryptophan, vitamins, and many secondary metabolites such as folates, ubiquinone and naphthoquinone [77]. The shikimate pathway takes place in the chloroplasts of green plants. The killing action of the herbicide requires that the plant be growing and exposed to light.

GM crops modified to be tolerant to Monsanto's formulation of glyphosate, called "Roundup Ready™," are modified with two main genes. One gene imparts reduced sensitivity to glyphosate and the other enables the plant to degrade glyphosate. The expression of both genes is directed to the chloroplasts, the site of the herbicide activity, by adding the coding sequences of a plant-derived "transit peptide."

The first gene encodes a bacteria-derived version of the plant enzyme involved in the shikimate biochemical pathway. Unlike the plant enzyme, which is sensitive to glyphosate, resulting in suppression of growth or death of the plant, the bacterial enzyme is insensitive to glyphosate. The second gene, also bacterial, codes for an enzyme that degrades glyphosate, and its coding sequence has been altered to enhance glyphosate-degrading activity.

The shikimate-chorismate pathway is not found in humans and mammals, and therefore represents a novel target; though it is present in a variety of microorganisms. However, glyphosate acts by preventing the binding of the metabolite, phosphoenol pyruvate (PEP), to the enzyme site [78]. PEP is a central metabolite present in all organisms, including humans. Glyphosate, therefore, has the potential to disrupt many important enzyme systems that utilize PEP, including energy metabolism and the synthesis of key membrane lipids required in nerve cells.

Glyphosate is the most frequent cause of complaints and poisoning in the UK [79]. Suicide attempts have been successful with as little as 100 milliliters of a 10 to 20% solution. Widespread disturbances of many body systems have been reported after exposures at normal use levels. These include balance disorders; vertigo; reduced cognitive capacity; seizures; impaired vision, smell, hearing and taste; headaches; drops in blood pressure; bodywide twitches and tics; muscle paralysis; peripheral neuropathy; loss of gross and fine motor skills; excessive sweating; and severe fatigue [80].

An epidemiological study in Ontario farm populations showed that glyphosate exposure nearly doubled the risk of late spontaneous abortion [81]. Children born to users of glyphosate were found to have elevated neurobehavioral defects [82]. Glyphosate caused retarded development of the fetal skeleton in laboratory rats [83].

Other experimental and animal studies suggest that glyphosate inhibits the synthesis of steroids [84], and is genotoxic in mammals [85, 86], fish [87, 88] and frogs [89, 90]. Field-dose exposure of earthworms caused at least 50% mortality and significant intestinal damage among surviving worms [91]. A recent paper reported that Roundup™ caused cell division dysfunction that may be linked to human cancers [92].

As reviewed in reference 76, the nitrogen-fixing symbiont in transgenic and nontransgenic soya is sensitive to glyphosate, and early application of glyphosate led to decreased crop biomass and nitrogen. Glyphosate application at elevated temperature (around 35°C) to Roundup Ready™ soya resulted in meristem damage, which is related to increased transport of the herbicide to the meristem.

Glyphosate application in conventional weed control led to the destruction and local extinction of endangered plant species. In forest ecosystems, it reduces bryophytes and lichens significantly.

Glyphosate treatment of bean seedlings resulted in short-term increases in dampening-off pathogens in treated soil.

Glyphosate application to control invasive species along tidal flats gave unexpected secondary effects. After spraying, the herbicide in sediment declined by 88%, while in the target perennial grass, the herbicide increased 591%, and was stored in the rhizomes. Glyphosate persists in soil and groundwater and was found in well water in sites adjacent to sprayed areas.

There is a wealth of published scientific studies showing that the massive increase in use of glyphosate in conjunction with GM crops poses a significant threat to human and animal health as well as to the environment.

8

Horizontal Gene Transfer

Horizontal Gene Transfer and Epidemics

Horizontal gene transfer, the direct transfer of genetic material into the genomes of organisms, whether of the same or totally unrelated species, is by far the most serious safety issue that is unique to genetic engineering [93].

The world has been whipped up into hysteria over terrorist attacks and "weapons of mass destruction" since September 11, 2001. Governments want to ban publication of sensitive scientific research results, and a group of major life sciences editors and authors has concurred. Some scientists even suggest an international body to police research and publication [65].

But few have acknowledged that genetic engineering itself is inherently dangerous, as first pointed out by the pioneers of genetic engineering in the Asilomar Declaration in the mid-1970s, and as some of us have been reminding the public and policy-makers more recently [94, 95].

But what caught the attention of the mainstream media was the report in January 2001 of how researchers in Australia "accidentally" created a deadly mouse virus that killed all its victims in the course of manipulating a harmless virus. "Disaster in the making: An engineered mouse virus leaves us one step away from the ultimate bioweapon," was the headline in the *New Scientist* article. The editorial showed even less restraint: "The genie is out, biotech has just sprung a nasty surprise. Next time, it could be catastrophic."

This, and the current SARS epidemic, remind us that horizontal gene transfer and recombination create new viruses and bacteria that cause diseases, and if genetic engineering does anything, it is to greatly enhance the scope and tendency for horizontal gene transfer and recombination.

Genetic Engineering Enhances the Scope and Tendency for Horizontal Gene Transfer

In the first place, genetic engineering involves the rampant recombination of genetic material from widely diverse sources that would otherwise have very little opportunity to mix and recombine in nature. Some newer techniques, for example, "DNA shuffling" [96, 97] will create, in a matter of minutes, millions of new recombinants in the laboratory that have never existed in billions of years of evolution. There is no limit to the sources of DNA that can be shuffled in this way.

In the second place, disease-causing viruses and bacteria and their genetic material are the predominant materials and tools of genetic engineering, as much as for the intentional creation of bio-weapons. And this includes antibiotic-resistant genes that make infections more difficult to treat.

And finally, the artificial constructs created by genetic engineering are designed to cross species barriers and to jump into genomes (i.e., to further enhance and speed up horizontal gene transfer and recombination) now acknowledged to be *the* major route to creating new disease agents, possibly much more important than point mutations which change isolated bases in the DNA.

Add to that the inherent instability of transgenic DNA mentioned earlier, which makes it more likely to break and recombine, and we begin to realize why we don't need bioterrorists when we have genetic engineers.

9

The CaMV 35S Promoter

"Recombination Hotspot"

Some transgenic constructs are less stable than others, such as those containing the cauliflower mosaic virus (CaMV) 35S promoter. The CaMV infects plants of the cabbage family. One of its promoters, the 35S promoter, has been widely used in GM crops since the beginning of plant genetic engineering, before some of its worrying features came to light. The most serious is its possession of a "recombination hotspot," where it tends to recombine with other DNA; although definitive evidence for that did not appear until much later.

Since the early 1990s, major doubts have arisen over the safety of viral genes incorporated into GM crops to make crops resistant to viral attack. Many of the viral genes tended to recombine with other viruses to generate new, and at times superinfectious, viruses.

In 1999, definitive evidence for the recombination hotspot in the CaMV 35S promoter came from work published independently by two research groups. This was highly significant in view of the findings of Ewen and Pusztai reviewed earlier, suggesting that the damage to young rats fed GM potatoes could be due to the transformation process itself or to the transgenic construct.

Ho et al. reviewed the safety implications of the CaMV 35S promoter, pointing out that its recombination hotspot is flanked by multiple motifs known to be involved in recombination, which are similar to other recombination hotspots, including the borders of the *Agrobacterium T-DNA* vector most frequently used in making transgenic plants. The suspected mechanism of recombination—double-stranded DNA breaks followed by repair—requires little or no DNA sequence homologies, and recombination between viral transgenes and infecting viruses has been amply demonstrated. In addition, the CaMV 35S promoter functions efficiently in all plants, as well as green algae, yeast and *E. coli*. It has a modular structure, with parts common to, and interchangeable with, promoters of many other plant and animal viruses.

These findings suggested that transgenic constructs with the CaMV 35S promoter might be especially unstable and prone to horizontal gene transfer and recombination, with all the attendant hazards: gene mutations due to random insertion; cancer; reactivation of dormant viruses and generation of new viruses, some of which could account for the observations described by Ewen and Pusztai [44, 46, 48, 51].

When Ho et al.'s paper [98] was accepted for publication, the journal *Microbial Ecology in Health and Disease* put out a press release on its Web site, labeling it a "hot topic." Within a day, someone by the name of Klaus Amman appeared to have organized at least nine critiques that rebounded around the Internet, ranging from the abusive and condescending to the relatively moderate. It later transpired that Klaus Amman is a key player in establishing (or, as we perceive, undermining) biosafety standards on the international scene, and holds many posts in organizations funded by the biotech industry.

Ho et al. answered all the criticisms in a paper that was circulated on the Internet, and subsequently was published in the same scientific journal. The critics have failed to respond to this day.

Unfortunately, the most outrageous and abusive remarks were incorporated into one "analysis" piece written by an editor of *Nature Biotechnology* under "Business and regulatory news" [99]. That "analysis," concocted entirely of hearsay and opinions, contained such defamatory, libelous statements that the journal had to give Ho et al. a right to reply when challenged. The reply was eventually published several months later [100] (along with the editor's "apology" that he had failed to cite their rebuttal), but was actually another attack on them. This time, *Nature Biotechnology* refused to let them reply.

All of the substantive scientific criticisms eventually turned up in a paper published in the journal where the original paper appeared, coauthored by Roger Hull and Phil Dale, a member of the UK Advisory Committee on Novel Foods and Processes (ACNFP) [101]. Their main criticisms boiled down to the following.

First, people have been eating virus-infected cabbage and cauliflower for many years without harm, so why should they worry about the CaMV 35S promoter?

Second, plants are already loaded with pararetroviral sequences, not unlike CaMV, so why should there be any risks?

The criticisms were thoroughly rebutted in a paper that was longer than the original, which appeared in the same journal soon afterwards [102]. And no further response followed. In fact, critics were careful never to mention the rebuttal.

It was pointed out, among other things, that people have *not* been eating CaMV 35S promoter plucked from its natural genetic and evolutionary context and incorporated into transgenic DNA.

The fact that plants are "loaded" with pararetroviral sequences similar to CaMV and other potentially mobile elements can only make things worse. Pararetroviruses are viruses that use reverse transcriptase, but do not depend on integrating into the host genome for replication. Pararetroviruses include a family that contains the human pathogen, hepatitis B virus. The CaMV 35S promoter could activate dormant viruses like hepatitis B, which was also known to have integrated into some human genomes and appeared to be associated with the disease.

Most, if not all, of the elements integrated into the genome would have been "tamed" in the course of evolution and therefore are no longer mobile. But integration of transgenic constructs containing the 35S promoter may mobilize the elements. The elements may in turn provide helper-functions to destabilize the transgenic DNA, and may also serve as substrates for recombination to generate more exotic invasive elements.

Evidence has since emerged that integration of foreign genes into the genome associated with the genetic modification can indeed activate transposons and proviral sequences, leading to destabilization of the genome [103]. So Ho et al. were not wide off the mark.

In the course of debating with the critics, Ho and his coworkers found even more damning evidence [104]. It turns out that although the CaMV virus infects only plants in the cabbage family, its 35S promoter is promiscuously active in species across the living world, not just bacteria, algae, fungi and plants, but also animal and human cells, as they discovered in a scientific paper dating back to 1990. Plant geneticists who have incorporated the CaMV 35S promoter into practically all GM crops now grown commercially were apparently unaware of that and are still not admitting to it in public.

The UK Advisory Committee on Releases to the Environment (ACRE) has no excuse for omitting the information in its latest report [105] reiterating "no evidence of harm," as Ho has drawn attention to it many times, both in written submissions and in oral evidence presented at several open hearings. Behind the scenes, however, the CaMV 35S promoter has been quietly withdrawn. It no longer appears in most of the GM crops under development.

The controversy surrounding the transgenic contamination of Mexican landraces is not so much that the contamination had occurred, rather, it is the possibility that, because the transgenic constructs were unstable, they could be, according to a critic [106], "fragmenting and promiscuously scattering throughout genomes." All the transgenic maize constructs that might have been responsible for the contamination contained the CaMV 35S promoter, which was why the promoter could be used to test for transgenic contamination. Such fragmentation and scattering of unstable DNA throughout the genome are known to activate dormant proviruses and transposons (see above), causing DNA rearrangements, deletions, translocations and other disturbances, which could destabilize the genomes of the landraces, driving the landraces toward extinction.

10

Transgenic DNA Is
More Likely to Spread

Transgenic DNA Versus Natural DNA

Transgenic DNA is different from natural DNA in many respects, all of which contribute to its increased propensity for horizontal transfer into genomes of unrelated organisms, where it may also recombine with new genes [93].

Transgenic DNA is more likely to spread horizontally

* Transgenic DNA often contains new combinations of genetic material that have never existed.
* Transgenic DNA has been designed to jump into genomes.
* The unnatural gene constructs tend to be structurally unstable and hence prone to break and join up or recombine with other genes.
* The mechanisms that enable foreign gene constructs to jump into the genome enable them to jump out again and reinsert at another site or in another genome. For example, the enzyme integrase, which catalyzes the insertion of viral DNA into the host genome, also functions as a *dis*integrase, catalyzing the reverse reaction. These integrases belong to a superfamily of similar enzymes that are present in all genomes, from viruses and bacteria to higher plants and animals. Recombinases of transposons are similar.
* The borders of the most commonly used vector for transgenic plants, the *T-DNA* of *Agrobacterium*, are recombination hotspots (sites that tend to break and join). In addition, a recombination hotspot is also associated with the cauliflower

mosaic virus (CaMV) promoter and many terminators (genetic signals for ending transcription), which means that the whole or parts of the integrated DNA will have an increased propensity for secondary horizontal gene transfer and recombination.

- Recent evidence indicates that foreign gene constructs tend to integrate at recombination hotspots in the genome, which, again, would tend to increase the chances of transgenic DNA *dis*integrating and transferring horizontally.

- Transgenic DNA often has other genetic signals, such as *origins of replication* left over from the plasmid vector. These are also recombination hotspots, and, in addition, can enable the transgenic DNA to be replicated independently as a plasmid that is readily transferred horizontally among bacteria.

- The metabolic stress on the host organism due to the continuous overexpression of the foreign genes linked to aggressive promoters, such as the CaMV 35S promoter, will also increase the instability of the transgenic DNA, thereby facilitating horizontal gene transfer.

- Transgenic DNA is typically a mosaic of DNA sequences from many different species and their genetic parasites; these homologies mean that it will be more prone to recombine with, and successfully transfer to, the genomes of many species as well as their genetic parasites. Homologous recombination typically occurs at one thousand to one million times the frequency of nonhomologous recombination.

Evidence that Transgenic DNA Is Different

There has been only one experiment ever carried out to test the hypothesis that transgenes are the same (or not the same) as mutants induced by conventional means (mutagenesis), such as exposure to X-rays and chemical mutagens, which cause changes in the base sequence of DNA.

Bergelson and colleagues [107] obtained a mutant for herbicide tolerance by conventional mutagenesis in a laboratory strain of *Arabidopsis* and created transgenic lines by introducing the mutant gene, spliced into a vector, into host plant cells.

They then compared the rate at which transgenic and non-transgenic mutant plants spread the herbicide-tolerance trait to normal, wild-type plants grown nearby. They found that the transgenes from transgenic plants were up to 30 times more likely to escape and spread than the same gene obtained by mutagenesis. The results are difficult to explain in terms of ordinary cross-pollination. Was it because introducing the transgene by means of a vector led to all kinds of unexpected effects? Did the transgenic plants produce more pollen, or more viable pollen? Was the pollen from transgenic plants more attractive to bees?

Another possibility for the increased spread of transgenes is horizontal gene transfer, via insects visiting the plants for pollen and nectar, or simply feeding on the sap or other parts of successive transgenic and wild-type plants. Bergelson said they had no evidence for horizontal gene transfer, but could not rule it out. They have not gone on to investigate that possibility.

Regardless of the manner in which the transgenes had spread, the experiment did demonstrate that transgenic DNA does not behave in the same way as nontransgenic DNA.

11

Horizontal Transfer
of Transgenic DNA

Experiments Demonstrating Horizontal Transfer of Transgenic DNA

Horizontal transfer of transgenes and antibiotic-resistant marker genes from genetically engineered crop plants into soil bacteria and fungi had been demonstrated in the laboratory by the mid-1990s. Transfer of transgenes to fungi was achieved simply by growing the fungi with the GM plant, and transfer to bacteria was achieved by applying total DNA from the GM plant to cultures of bacteria.

By the late 1990s, successful transfers of a kanamycin-resistance marker gene to the soil bacterium *Acinetobacter* were obtained with total DNA extracted from homogenized leaves in a range of transgenic plants [108]: *Solanum tuberosum* (potato), *Nicotiana tabacum* (tobacco), *Beta vulgaris* (sugar beet), *Brassica napus* (oilseed rape), and *Lycopersicon esculentum* (tomato). It was estimated that about 2500 copies of the kanamycin-resistance genes (from the same number of plant cells) were sufficient to successfully transform one bacterium, despite the fact that there was a 6×10^6-fold excess of plant DNA present. Positive results of horizontal gene transfer in this system were obtained even with just 100 microliters of ground-up plant leaf added to the bacteria.

Obfuscation and Misrepresentation

From the beginning obfuscation and misrepresentation reigned supreme. Despite the misleading title in a paper by Schluter, Futterer and Potrykus, which states that horizontal gene transfer in their experiment "occurs, if at all, at an extremely low-frequency" [109], the data demonstrated a high frequency of gene transfer of 5.8×10^{-2} per recipient bacterium under optimum conditions.

Nevertheless, the authors proceeded to calculate a theoretical gene transfer frequency of 2.0 x 10^{-17}, or close to zero, under extrapolated "'natural conditions." This was done by assuming that different factors acted independently, and by inventing the "natural conditions," which are largely unknown and unpredictable—even though the authors themselves admitted that synergistic effects from combinations of factors cannot be ruled out.

This paper was subsequently widely cited as illustrating that horizontal gene transfer does not happen.

Field Experiment Provides *Prima Facie* Evidence

In 1999 researchers in Germany [110] had already reported the first, and still only, field-monitoring experiment in the world that provided *prima facie* evidence that transgenic DNA had transferred from the GM-sugar-beet plant debris to bacteria in the soil. Ho circulated a detailed review of this evidence and duly submitted it to the UK government's science advisors. They dismissed that evidence, and worse, cited it as evidence that horizontal gene transfer did not occur.

DNA not only persists in the external environment, both in the soil and in water, it is not broken down sufficiently quickly in the digestive system to prevent transgenic DNA from transferring to microorganisms resident in the gut of animals.

Transgenic DNA Transfer in the Mouth

Such transfer could start in the mouth. Mercer et al. reported in 1999 [111] that a genetically engineered plasmid had a 6–25% chance of surviving intact after 60 minutes of exposure to human saliva. Moreover, the partially degraded plasmid DNA was capable of transforming *Streptococcus gordonii*, one of the bacteria that normally live in the human mouth and pharynx. The frequency of transformation dropped exponentially with time, but it was still significant after 10 minutes. Human saliva actually contains factors that promote transformation in bacteria resident in the mouth.

This research was done in the test tube, and the authors clearly stated that "further investigations are needed to establish whether transformation of oral bacteria can occur at significant frequencies *in vivo*." However, no such studies have been carried out since then, which is difficult to understand since *the original research had been commissioned by the UK government as part of the Novel Foods Program.*

Another group in Leeds University, however, got a grant from the then newly established Food Standards Agency (FSA) to investigate the possibility of horizontal gene transfer in the stomachs of ruminants [112], where food remains for long periods of time. The researchers found that transgenic DNA was rapidly broken down in the fluids from the rumen and the silage, but that, nevertheless, horizontal transfer could take place before the transgenic DNA was completely degraded.

They also found that transgenic DNA was very slow to break down in saliva; therefore, the mouth could be a major site for horizontal gene transfer. This confirmed the results obtained by Mercer et al. [111]. But, once again, no follow-up work was done in live animals. Was it a case of avoiding doing the obvious experiments for fear of finding positive results that would be more difficult to dismiss?

Transfer of Transgenic DNA Through the Wall of the Intestine and the Placenta

There's more to the scope of horizontal gene transfer as revealed in the existing scientific literature. Döerfler's group in Germany have carried out a series of experiments on the fate of foreign DNA in food beginning in the early 1990s.

They fed mice DNA, either isolated from the bacteria virus M13 or as the cloned gene for the green fluorescent protein inserted into a plasmid. They found that a small, albeit significant percentage of the viral and plasmid DNA not only escaped complete degradation in the gut but could pass through the wall of the intestine into the bloodstream to get into some white blood cells, the spleen and liver cells, and become incorporated into the mouse cell genome [113]. When fed to pregnant mice, the foreign DNA could be found in some cells of the fetuses and the newborn animals, showing that it had gone through the placenta [114].

This work underlines the hazards of all kinds of naked DNA, including viral genomes created by the genetic engineering industry, that Norwegian virologist and science advisor to the Norwegian government, Terje Traavik [115], and others [94, 95] have drawn attention to.

In a paper published in 1998, Döerfler and Schubbert stated [114]: "The consequences of foreign DNA uptake for mutagenesis [generating mutations] and oncogenesis [causing cancer] have not yet been investigated." The relevance of this remark is striking with regard to the cancer cases identified among the recipients of gene therapy in the latter part of 2002 [116]. It makes the point that exposures to transgenic DNA carry the same risks, regardless of whether it is from gene therapy or from GM foods. Gene therapy is just the genetic modification of human beings and uses constructs very similar to those for the genetic modification of plants and animals.

Avoidance of Definitive Experiments

In a report published in 2001 [117], the fate of ordinary soybean DNA from soybean leaves was compared with that of transgenic plasmid DNA. It confirmed earlier findings. Transgenic plasmid DNA invaded the cells of many tissues.

But like most of the research projects reviewed, this one too, seemed to stop short of attempting to obtain clearer, definitive results, which could easily have been accomplished by feeding mice transgenic soya, and monitoring for the fate of both the transgenic DNA and the plant's own DNA. That would have gone some way to settle the issue Ho and Cummins have repeatedly raised: that transgenic DNA may be more invasive of cells and genomes than natural DNA.

Indeed, as Ewen points out [44], the possibility cannot be excluded that feeding GM products, such as maize, to animals also carries risks. Cow's milk may contain GM derivatives and even a fillet of steak may contain active GM material, as DNA is extraordinarily stable and is often not destroyed by heat. DNA has even been recovered recently from soil sediments 300,000 to 400,000 years old [118]. Professor Alan Cooper, the lead researcher of Oxford University, on his recent visit to New Zealand, is reported to have said [119], "The ability of DNA to persist in soils for so long was completely underestimated . . . and illustrates how little we know," and "a great deal more research is needed before we could predict the effect of releasing GE plants."

Transgenic DNA in Food Transferred to Bacteria in the Human Gut

The UK government eventually commissioned research to look for horizontal gene transfer into bacteria in the gut of human volunteers and found positive results.

The research in question is the final part of the UK FSA project on evaluating the risks of GMOs in human foods [120].

The transfer of transgenic DNA to bacteria in the human gut is not at all unexpected. We already know from previous research reviewed here that DNA persists in the gut and that bacteria can readily take up foreign DNA. Why had our regulators waited so long to commission the research? And when they did, the scientists appeared to have designed the experiment so as to stack the odds heavily against finding a positive result [121].

For example, the method for detecting transgenic DNA depended on amplifying a small part—180bp—of the entire transgenic DNA insert, which was at least ten or twenty times as long. So, any other fragment of the insert would not be detected, nor would a fragment that did not overlap the whole 180bp amplified, or that had been rearranged. The chance of obtaining a positive result is 5% at best, and likely to be much, much less. *Thus, a negative finding with this detection method most probably would not indicate the absence of transgenic DNA.*

Despite all of this, they still found a positive result, which the FSA immediately dismissed and obfuscated. It was reported that the FSA claimed "the findings had been assessed by several Government experts who had ruled that humans were not at risk." In a statement on its Web site, the FSA said that the study had concluded it is "extremely unlikely" that GM genes can end up in the gut of people who eat them.

Agrobacterium Vector a Vehicle for Gene Escape

That is not all. Recent evidence strongly suggests that the most common method of creating transgenic plants may also serve as a ready route for horizontal gene transfer [122, 123].

Agrobacterium tumefaciens, the soil bacterium that causes crown gall disease, has been developed as a major gene transfer vector for making transgenic plants. Foreign genes are typically spliced into the *T-DNA* part of a plasmid of *A. tumefaciens* called Ti (tumor-inducing), which ends up integrated into the genome of the plant cell that subsequently develops into a tumor. That much has been known at least since 1980.

But further investigations revealed that the process whereby *Agrobacterium* injects *T-DNA* into plant cells strongly resembles *conjugation*, or mating between bacterial cells.

Conjugation, mediated by certain bacterial plasmids, requires a sequence called the origin of transfer (*oriT*) on the DNA that's transferred. All the other functions can be supplied from unlinked sources, referred to as "trans-acting functions" (or *tra*). Thus, "disabled" plasmids, with no trans-acting functions, can nevertheless be transferred by "helper" plasmids that carry genes coding for the *tra* functions. That is the basis of a complicated vector system involving *Agrobacterium T-DNA*, which has been used for creating numerous transgenic plants.

However, it was soon discovered that the left and right borders of the *T-DNA* are similar to *oriT*, and can be replaced by it. Furthermore, the disarmed *T-DNA*, lacking the *tra* functions (*virulence* genes that contribute to disease), can be helped by similar genes belonging to many other pathogenic bacteria. It seems that the trans-kingdom gene transfer of *Agrobacterium* and the conjugative systems of bacteria are both involved in transporting macromolecules—not just DNA, but protein as well.

That means transgenic plants created by the *T-DNA* vector system have a ready route for horizontal gene escape, via *Agrobacterium*, helped by the ordinary conjugative mechanisms of many other bacteria that cause diseases, and which are present in the environment.

In fact, the possibility that *Agrobacterium* can serve as a vehicle for horizontal gene escape was first raised in 1997 in a study sponsored by the UK Government [124], which reported it was extremely difficult to get rid of the *Agrobacterium* in the vector system after transformation. Treatment with an armory of antibiotics and repeated subculture over 13 months failed to get rid of the bacterium. Furthermore, 12.5% of the *Agrobacterium* remaining still contained the binary vector (*T-DNA* and helper plasmid), and were therefore fully capable of transforming other plants. This research was later published in a scientific journal [125].

Several other observations make gene escape via *Agrobacterium* even more likely. *Agrobacterium* not only transfers genes into plant cells, there is a possibility for retrotransfer of DNA from the plant cell to *Agrobacterium* [126].

High rates of gene transfer are associated with a plant's root system and the germinating seed, where conjugation is most likely [127]. There, *Agrobacterium* could multiply and transfer transgenic DNA to other bacteria, as well as to the next crop to be planted. These possibilities have yet to be investigated empirically.

Finally, *Agrobacterium* attaches to and genetically transforms several human cell lines [128]. In stable transformed HeLa cells (a human cell line derived originally from a cancer patient), the integration of *T-DNA* occurred at the right border, exactly as would happen when it is transferred into a plant cell genome. This suggests that *Agrobacterium* transforms human cells by a mechanism similar to that which it uses for transforming plants cells.

12

Hazards of Horizontal
Gene Transfer

A Summary
As clarified in the earlier chapters, hazards that could arise from the horizontal transfer of transgenic DNA are unique to genetic engineering. They are summarized below.

Potential hazards of horizontal gene transfer from genetic engineering

- Generation of new cross-species viruses that cause disease.
- Generation of new bacteria that cause disease.
- Spread of drug- and antibiotic-resistant genes among the viral and bacterial pathogens, making infections untreatable.
- Random insertion into genomes of cells, resulting in harmful effects, including cancer.
- Reactivation and recombination with dormant viruses (present in all genomes) to generate infectious viruses.
- Spread of dangerous new genes and gene constructs that have never existed.
- Destabilization of genomes into which transgenes have transferred.
- Multiplication of ecological impacts due to all of the above.

Experiments that Appear to Have Been Avoided So Far

These critiques have been communicated to ACRE and ACNFP, together with a series of obvious experiments that the FSA should commission, in a paper tabled at an open meeting organized by ACNFP [129]. These are described in a slightly revised form below.

Missing experiments on the safety of GM food and crops

The following are some definitive experiments that would inform on the safety of GM food and crops. They seem to have been intentionally avoided so far.

1. Feeding experiments similar to those carried out by Pusztai's team, using well-characterized transgenic soya and/or maize meal feed, with appropriate, unbiased monitoring for transgenic DNA in the feces, blood and blood cells, and post-mortem histological examinations that include tracking transfer of transgenic DNA into the genome of cells. As an added control, nontransgenic DNA from the same GM-feed sample should also be monitored. In addition; the role of the CaMV 35S promoter in producing the "growth factor-like" effects in young rats should be investigated.

2. Feeding trials on human volunteers using well-characterized transgenic soya and/or maize meal feed, with appropriate, unbiased monitoring for transgenic DNA and horizontal gene transfer in the mouth and in the feces, blood and blood cells. As an added control, nontransgenic DNA from the same GM-feed sample should also be monitored.

3. Investigation on the stability of transgenic plants in successive generations of growth, especially those containing the CaMV 35S promoter, using appropriate quantitative molecular techniques.

4. Full molecular characterization of all transgenic lines to establish uniformity and genetic stability of the transgenic DNA insert(s), and comparison with the original data supplied by the biotech company to gain approval for field trials or for commercial release.

5. Tests on all transgenic plants created by the *Agrobacterium T-DNA* vector system for the persistence of the bacteria and the vectors. The soil in which the transgenic plants have been grown should be monitored for gene escape to soil bacteria. The potential for horizontal gene transfer to the next crop via the germinating seed and root system should be carefully monitored.

13

Conclusions to
Parts 1 and 2

Our extensive review of the evidence has convinced us that GM crops are neither needed nor wanted, that they have failed to deliver their promises and, instead, are posing escalating problems on the farm. There is no realistic possibility for GM and non-GM agriculture to coexist, as evident from the level and extent of transgenic contamination that has already occurred, even in a country like Mexico where an official moratorium has been in place since 1998.

More importantly, GM crops are unacceptable because they are by no means safe. They have been introduced without the necessary safeguards and safety assessments through a deeply flawed regulatory system based on a principle of "substantial equivalence" that is aimed at expediting product approval rather than serious safety assessment.

Despite the lack of data on safety tests of GM foods, the available findings already raise cause for concerns over the safety of the transgenic process itself that are not being addressed.

At the same time, gene products introduced into food and other crops as biopesticides, accounting for 25% of all GM crops worldwide, are now found to be strong immunogens and allergens, and dangerous pharmaceuticals and vaccines are being introduced into food crops in open field trials.

Under the guise of transgene containment, crops have been engineered with "suicide genes" that make plants male-sterile. In reality, these crops spread both herbicide-tolerant genes and male-sterile suicide genes via pollen, which could lead to potentially devastating consequences on agricultural and natural biodiversity.

About 75% of the GM crops planted worldwide are tolerant to one or the other of two broad-spectrum herbicides, glufosinate ammonium and glyphosate. Both are systemic metabolic poisons expected to have a wide range of harmful effects on humans and other living organisms, and these effects have now been confirmed.

Glufosinate ammonium is linked to neurological, respiratory, gastrointestinal and hematological toxicities, and birth defects in humans and mammals.

Glyphosate is the most frequent cause of complaints and poisoning in the UK, and disturbances of many body functions have been reported after exposures at normal use levels. Glyphosate exposure nearly doubled the risk of late spontaneous abortion, and children born to users of glyphosate had elevated neurobehavioral defects. Glyphosate caused retarded development of the fetal skeleton in laboratory rats. It inhibits the synthesis of steroids, and is genotoxic in mammals, fish and frogs. Field-dose exposure of earthworms caused at least 50% mortality and significant intestinal damage among surviving worms. Roundup™ causes cell division dysfunction that may be linked to human cancers.

These known effects are sufficient to call a halt to all uses of both herbicides.

By far the most insidious dangers of genetic engineering are inherent to the process itself, which greatly enhances the scope and probability of horizontal gene transfer and recombination, the main route to creating viruses and bacteria that cause disease epidemics.

Newer techniques, such as DNA shuffling are allowing geneticists to create in a matter of minutes in the laboratory millions of recombinant viruses that have never existed. Disease-causing viruses and bacteria and their genetic material are the predominant materials and tools of genetic engineering, as much as for the intentional creation of bioweapons.

There is already experimental evidence that transgenic DNA from plants has been taken up by bacteria in the soil and in the gut of human volunteers. Antibiotic-resistance marker genes can spread from transgenic food to pathogenic bacteria, making infections very difficult to treat.

Transgenic DNA is known to survive digestion in the gut and to jump into the genome of mammalian cells, raising the possibility for triggering cancer.

Evidence suggests that transgenic constructs with the CaMV 35S promoter, present in most GM crops, might be especially unstable and prone to horizontal gene transfer and recombination, with all the attendant hazards: gene mutations due to random insertion, cancer, reactivation of dormant viruses and generation of new viruses.

There has been a history of misrepresentation and suppression of scientific evidence, especially on horizontal gene transfer.

Key experiments failed to be performed, or were performed badly and then misrepresented. Many experiments failed to be followed up, including investigations on whether the CaMV 35S promoter is responsible for the "growth factor-like" effects observed in young rats fed GM potatoes.

For all of these reasons, GM crops should be firmly rejected as a viable option for the future of agriculture.

Part 3: The Manifold Benefits of Sustainable Agriculture

14

Why Sustainable Agriculture?

Alternative Agriculture Needed

"Modern" agriculture is characterized by extensive, large-scale monoculture and depends on high chemical inputs and intensive mechanization.

Although productive as defined by the one-dimensional measure of "yield" of a single crop, its overreliance on chemical pesticides, herbicides and synthetic fertilizers comes with a string of negative impacts on health and the environment: health risks to farm workers, harmful chemical residues on food, reduced biodiversity, deterioration of soil and water quality, and increased risks of crop disease. "Modern" monoculture also often marginalizes small farmers, particularly those in developing countries, who are the majority of farmers worldwide. GM crops, now thrown into the package, are threatening further health and environmental hazards (see Part 2).

Many Different Sustainable Agricultural Practices

In contrast, sustainable agricultural approaches place the emphasis on a diversity of local natural resources, and on local autonomy of farmers to decide what they will grow and how they can improve their crops and livelihood.

Agriculture is sustainable when it is ecologically sound, economically viable, socially just, culturally appropriate, humane and based on a holistic approach. A brief summary of key criteria, as elaborated by Pretty and Hine [130], is presented on page 61.

Sustainable agricultural approaches may come under many names—agroecology, sustainable agriculture, organic agriculture, ecological agriculture, biological agriculture—but have these criteria in common.

For example, organic farming largely excludes synthetic pesticides, herbicides and fertilizers. Instead, it is an ecosystem approach that manages ecological and biological processes, such as food-web relations, nutrient cycling, maintaining soil fertility, natural pest control and diversifying crops and livestock. It relies on locally or farm-derived renewable resources, while remaining environmentally and ecologically viable.

While many in developed countries may be familiar with certified organic production, this is just the tip of the iceberg in terms of land managed organically but not certified as such.

De facto or noncertified organic farming is usually prevalent in resource-poor and/or agriculturally marginal regions where local populations have limited engagement with the cash economy [131]. Farmers here rely on local natural resources to maintain soil fertility and to combat pests and diseases. They have sophisticated systems of crop rotation, soil management, and pest and disease control, based on traditional knowledge.

Likewise, agroecology relies on technologies that are cheap, accessible, risk-averting and productive in marginal environments; that enhance ecological and human health; and that are culturally and socially acceptable [132]. It emphasizes biodiversity; nutrient recycling; synergy among crops, animals, soils and other biological components; as well as regeneration and conservation of resources. Agroecology relies on indigenous farming knowledge and incorporates low-input modern technologies to diversify production. The approach combines ecological principles and local resources in managing farming systems, providing an environmentally sound and affordable way for small farmers to intensify production in marginal areas.

These agroecological alternatives can solve the agricultural problems that GM crops claim to solve, but do so in a much more socially equitable and environmentally harmonious manner [3].

There are countless studies as well as scientific research papers documenting the successes and benefits of sustainable agricultural approaches, including those of organic farming, which have been reviewed recently by the FAO [133] and ISIS [134].

We summarize the evidence on some of the benefits of agroecology, sustainable agriculture and organic farming for the environment and health, as well as for food security and the social well-being of farmers and local communities. It makes the case for a comprehensive shift to these sustainable agriculture approaches in place of GM crops.

Sustainable agriculture

- Makes best use of nature's goods and services by integrating natural, regenerative processes (e.g., nutrient cycling, nitrogen fixation, soil regeneration and natural enemies of pests).
- Minimizes nonrenewable inputs (pesticides and fertilizers) that damage the environment or harm human health.
- Relies on the knowledge and skills of farmers, improving their self-reliance.
- Promotes and protects social capital—people's capacities to work together to solve problems.
- Depends on locally adapted practices to innovate in the face of uncertainty.
- Is multifunctional and contributes to public goods, such as clean water, wildlife, carbon sequestration in soils, flood protection and landscape quality.

15

Higher or Comparable Productivity and Yields

A Closer Look at Yields

Organic agriculture is often criticized for having lower yields compared to conventional monoculture. While that may be the case in industrialized countries, such comparisons are misleading because they discount the costs of conventional monoculture in degraded land, water, biodiversity and other ecological services on which sustainable food production depends [133].

And merely looking at yields for single crops—as critics often do—misses other indicators of sustainability and higher actual productivity per unit area, particularly with agroecological systems that often have a diverse mixture of crops, trees and animals together on the land [135] (see "Efficient, Profitable Production"). It is often possible to obtain the highest yield of a single crop by planting it alone—in a monoculture. But while a monoculture may allow for a high yield of one crop, it produces nothing else of use to the farmer [136].

In any case, because of the damage done by conventional farming, a transition period is usually required to restore the land for the full benefits of sustainable farming. After the system is restored, comparable or higher yields are obtained. With low-input, traditional agriculture, conversion to sustainable approaches is normally accompanied by immediately increased yields.

In fact, just reducing average farm size in most countries would stimulate increases in production far beyond the most optimistic biotech industry projections for GM crops. Small farms are more productive, more efficient, and contribute more to economic development than the large farms characteristic of conventional monoculture [136]. Small farmers are also better stewards of natural resources.

Research from around the world shows that smaller farms are from two to ten times more productive per hectare than larger farms, which tend to be inefficient, extensive monocultures. Yield increases are achieved by using technological approaches based on agro-ecological principles that emphasize diversity, synergy, recycling and integration; and social processes that emphasize community participation and empowerment. As average farm sizes are usually in the larger, more inefficient range, genuine land reform offers an opportunity to boost production while lessening poverty.

Outstanding Successes in Developing Countries

The success of sustainable agriculture has been concretely demonstrated in a review of 208 projects and initiatives from 52 countries [130]. Some 8.98 million farmers have adopted sustainable agriculture practices on 28.92 million hectares in Africa, Asia and Latin America.

Reliable data on yield changes in 89 projects show that farmers have achieved substantial increases in food production per hectare, about 50–100% for rain-fed crops, though considerably greater in a few cases, and 5–10% for irrigated crops (though generally starting from a higher absolute yield base). These projects included both certified and noncertified organic systems, and integrated as well as near-organic systems. In all cases where reliable data were available, there were increases in per hectare productivity for food crops and maintenance of existing yields for fiber [133].

Some specific examples of increased yields are as follows:

- Soil and water conservation in the drylands of Burkina Faso has transformed formerly degraded lands. The average family has shifted from a cereal deficit of 644 kg per year (equivalent to 6.5 months of food shortage) to producing an annual surplus of 153 kg.
- Through the Cheha Integrated Rural Development Project in Ethiopia, some 12,500 households have adopted sustainable agriculture, resulting in a 60% increase in crop yields.
- In Madagascar, a system of rice intensification has improved rice yields from some 2 t/ha to 5, 10, or 15 t/ha, without recourse to purchased inputs of pesticides or fertilizers.
- In Sri Lanka, some 55,000 households on about 33,000 ha have adopted sustainable agriculture, with substantial reductions in insecticide use. Yields have increased by 12–44% for rice and 7–44% for vegetables.

- 45,000 families in Honduras and Guatemala have increased crop yields from 400–600 kg/ha to 2000–2500 kg/ha using green manures, cover crops, contour grass strips, in-row tillage, rock bunds and animal manures.
- The states of Santa Caterina, Paraná and Rio Grande do Sol in southern Brazil have focused on soil and water conservation using contour grass barriers, contour plowing and green manures. Maize yields have risen by 67% from 3 to 5 t/ha, and soybeans by 68% from 2.8 to 4.7 t/ha.
- The high mountain regions of Bolivia are some of the most difficult areas in the world for growing crops. Despite this, farmers have increased potato yields by threefold, particularly by using green manures to enrich the soil.

Other case studies of organic and agroecological practices show dramatic increases in yields as well as benefits to soil quality, reduction in pests and diseases and general improvement in taste and nutritional content [131]. For example:

- In Brazil, use of green manures and cover crops increased maize yields by 20–250%.
- In Tigray, Ethiopia, yields of crops from composted plots were 3–5 times higher than those treated only with chemicals.
- Yield increases of 175% are reported from farms in Nepal adopting agroecological practices.
- In Peru, restoration of traditional Incan terracing has led to increases of 150% for a range of upland crops. Farmers are able to produce bumper crops despite floods, droughts and the lethal frosts common at altitudes of nearly 4000 meters [135].
- Projects in Senegal involving 2000 farmers promoted stall-fed livestock, composting systems, green manures, water harvesting systems and rock phosphate. Millet and peanut yields increased dramatically, by 75–195% and 75–165%, respectively. Because the soils have greater water-retaining capacity, yield fluctuations are less pronounced between high and low rainfall years.
- In Santa Catarina, Brazil, focus has been on soil and water conservation, using contour grass barriers, contour plowing and green manures. Some 60 different crop species, leguminous and nonleguminous, have been intercropped or planted during fallow periods. These have had major impact

on yields, soil quality, levels of biological activity and water-retaining capacity: maize and soybean yields have increased by 66%.

- In Honduras, soil conservation practices and organic fertilizers have tripled or quadrupled yields.

Planting the *mucuna* bean has improved crop yields on steep, easily eroded hillsides with depleted soils in Honduras [137]. Farmers first plant *mucuna*, which produces vigorous growth that suppresses weeds. When the beans are cut down, maize is planted in the resulting mulch. Subsequently, beans and maize are grown together. Very quickly, as the soil improves, yields are doubled, even tripled (see "Better Soils"). The reason: *mucuna* produces lots of organic material, creating rich, friable soils. It also produces its own fertilizer, fixing atmospheric nitrogen (N) and storing it in the ground for other plants.

This simple technology has also been adopted in Nicaragua, where more than 1000 peasants recovered degraded land in the San Juan watershed in just one year. These farmers have decreased the use of chemical fertilizers from 1900 to 400 kilograms per hectare while increasing yields from 700 to 2000 kilograms per hectare. Their production costs are about 22% lower than that for farmers using chemical fertilizers and monocultures [135].

Phosphorus (P) is the most important nutrient (after N) that is most frequently deficient in soils of tropical Africa. Unlike N, P cannot get into the soil by biological fixation. Therefore, the availability of P from organic and inorganic sources is essential to maximize and sustain high crop-yield potential.

Studies in western Kenya compared the impact of organic and inorganic fertilizers [138]. The scientists concluded that reasonable maize yields could be achieved in smallholder systems if adequate amounts of high-quality organic materials were used as P sources.

Comparisons in Industrialized Countries

Organic farming also compares favorably against conventional monoculture in industrialized countries. A review of scientifically replicated research results from seven different U.S. universities and data from two research centers over ten years shows that yields from organic systems and conventional monoculture are comparable [139].

- Corn: With 69 total cropping seasons, organic yields were 94% of conventionally produced corn.

- Soybeans: Data from five states with 55 growing seasons showed organic yields were 94% of conventional yields.
- Wheat: Two institutions with 16 cropping years showed that organic wheat produced 97% of the conventional yields.
- Tomatoes: 14 years of comparative research on tomatoes showed no yield differences.

Vasilikiotis reviewed recent studies comparing the productivity of organic practices to conventional agriculture [140], including the Sustainable Agriculture Farming Systems (SAFS) and Rodale studies discussed below, and concluded that "organic farming methods can produce higher yields than conventional methods." Furthermore, "a worldwide conversion to organic has the potential to increase food production levels—not to mention reversing the degradation of agricultural soils—and increase soil fertility and health."

Results from the first 15 years of a long-term, large-scale experiment carried out by the Rodale Institute showed that after a transition period of four years, crops grown under organic systems (animal- and legume-based) yielded as much as and sometimes more than conventional crops [141]. Moreover, organic systems outproduced the conventional system when conditions were less than optimal, for example during drought (see "Better Soils").

Initial lower yields were attributed partly to inadequate availability of N, the time taken for soil microbial activity to stabilize (soils generally contained enough total N but not yet in a usable form) and heavier weed growth. These could be addressed by appropriate management and given time for the system to adjust to the shift to organic farming.

A four-year study, part of the larger, longer-term SAFS project at the University of California, Davis, compared conventional and alternative farming systems for tomatoes [142]. Results indicated that organic and low-input production gave comparable yields to conventional systems. N availability was the most important yield-limiting factor in organic systems, but could be addressed by appropriate management. Additional N, when associated with high carbon inputs, built up soil organic matter, enhancing long-term fertility. Eventually, soil organic-matter levels stabilized, requiring less N input.

Results from the first eight years of the SAFS project showed that the organic and low-input systems had yields comparable to the conventional systems in all crops tested—tomato, safflower, corn and bean—and, in some instances, the yields were higher than those of conventional systems [143]. Tomato yields in the organic system were lower in the first three years, but then caught up with the conventional system, overtaking it in the last year of the experiment (80 t/ha compared to 68 t/ha in 1996). Both organic and low-input systems increased soil organic carbon content and stored nutrients, both critical for long-term soil fertility. As soil organic-matter levels stabilized during the last two years of the experiment, resulting in more N availability, higher yields of organic crops were observed. The organic systems were found to be more profitable for both corn and tomatoes, mainly due to higher price premiums.

Another experiment compared organic and conventional potatoes and sweet corn over three years [144]. No differences in yield and vitamin C content of potatoes were found. While one variety of conventional corn outproduced the organic, there was no difference between conventional and organic in the yield of another variety, or in vitamin C or E contents of corn kernels. The results suggested that long-term application of composts produces higher soil fertility and comparable plant growth.

16

Better Soils

Soil Conservation

Most sustainable agricultural practices reduce soil erosion and improve soil physical structure, organic-matter content, water-holding capacity and nutrient balances. Soil fertility is maintained on existing lands and restored on degraded lands.

A powerful example is that of farmers along the Sahara's edge (in Nigeria, Niger, Senegal, Burkina Faso and Kenya), who farm productively without destroying soils, even in dryland areas. Integrated farming, mixed cropping and traditional soil and water conservation methods are increasing per-capita food production severalfold [145, 146].

Sustainable agricultural approaches help conserve and improve the farmers' most precious resource—the topsoil. To counter the problems of hardening, nutrient loss and erosion, organic farmers in the South are using trees, shrubs and legumes to stabilize and feed soil, dung and compost to provide nutrients, and terracing or check dams to prevent erosion and conserve groundwater [131].

Restoring Soil Fertility

Planting *mucuna* beans in Latin America has restored soil fertility on depleted soils [137]. *Mucuna* produces 100 tons of organic material per hectare, creating rich, friable soils in a few years. It produces its own fertilizer, fixing atmospheric N and storing it in the ground for use by other plants. As the soil improves, yields are doubled, even tripled.

One of the longest running agricultural trials on record (more than 150 years) is the Broadbalk experiment at Rothamsted Experimental Station. The trials compare a manure-based fertilizer farming system to a synthetic chemical fertilizer system. Wheat yields are, on average, slightly higher in organically fertilized plots than in plots receiving chemical fertilizers. More importantly, soil fertility, measured as soil organic matter and nitrogen levels, increased by 120% over 150 years in the organic plots, compared with only a 20% increase in chemically fertilized plots [147].

Another study compared ecological characteristics and productivity of 20 commercial farms in California [148]. Tomato yields were quite similar in organic and conventional farms. Insect pest damage was also comparable. Significant differences were found in soil health indicators such as N mineralization potential and microbial abundance and diversity, which were higher in the organic farms. N mineralization potential was three times greater in organic compared to conventional fields. The organic fields also had 28% more organic carbon. The increased soil health resulted in considerably lower disease incidence. Severity of the most prevalent disease in the study, tomato corky root disease, was significantly lower in the organic farms.

Improving Soil Ecology

The world's longest running experiment comparing organic and conventional farming pronounced the former a success [149, 150]. The 21-year Swiss study found that soils nourished with manure were more fertile and produced more crops for a given input of nitrogen or other fertilizer.

The biggest bonus was improved soil quality under organic cultivation. Organic soils had up to 3.2 times as much biomass and abundance of earthworms, twice as many arthropods (important predators and indicators of soil fertility) and 40% more mycorrhizal fungi colonizing plant roots. Mycorrhizal fungi help roots obtain more nutrients and water from the soil [151]. The increased diversity of microbial communities in organic soils transformed carbon from organic debris into biomass at lower energy costs, building up a higher microbial biomass. Hence a more diverse microbial community is more efficient in resource utilization. The enhanced soil fertility and higher biodiversity in organic soils is thought to reduce dependency on external inputs and provide long-term environmental benefits.

Field experiments conducted at three organic and three conventional vegetable farms in 1996–1997 examined the effects of synthetic fertilizers and alternative soil amendments, including compost [152]. Propagule densities of *Trichoderma* species (beneficial soil fungi that are biological control agents of plant-pathogenic fungi) and thermophilic microorganisms (a major constituent of which was Actinomycetes, which suppresses *Phytophthora*) were greater in organic soils. In contrast, densities of *Phytophthora* and *Pythium* (both plant pathogens) were lower in organic soils.

While the study recorded increased enteric bacteria in organic soils, the scientists stressed that this was not a problem, as survival rates in soil are minimal. (Critics of organic farming disingenuously point to the possible health effects of using manure. But untreated manure is *not* allowed in certified organic agriculture, and treated manure (known widely as compost) is safe—this is what is used in organic farming. Unlike conventional regimes (where untreated manure might be used), organic certification bodies inspect farms to ensure standards are met [153].)

Few significant differences in yields were observed between soils with alternative amendments and those with synthetic fertilizers, regardless of production system. In 1997, when all growers planted tomatoes, the yields were higher on farms with a history of organic production, regardless of soil-amendment type, due to the benefits of long-term organic amendments. Mineral concentrations were higher in organic soils, and soil quality in conventional farms was significantly improved by organic fertilizer. The researchers concluded that "the argument [of critics] that organic farming is equivalent to low yield farming is not supported by our data" (p.158).

Overall Improved Soil Quality: Averting Crop Failure During Drought

The 15-year study carried out by the Rodale Institute compared three maize/soybean agroecosystems [141, 154, 155]. One was a conventional system using mineral N fertilizer and pesticides. The other two systems were managed organically. One was manure-based, where grasses and legumes, grown as part of a crop rotation, were fed to cattle. The manure provided N for maize production. The other system did not have livestock, but leguminous cover crops were incorporated into soil as a source of N.

Organic techniques were found to significantly improve soil quality, as measured by structure, total soil organic matter (a measure of soil fertility) and biological activity [141]. The improved soil structure created a better root-zone environment for growing plants and allowed the soil to better absorb and retain moisture. Apart from the benefit during low-rainfall periods, it reduced the potential for erosion in severe storms.

Organic soils showed a higher level of microbial activity and a greater diversity of microorganisms. Such long-term changes in the soil community could promote plant health and might positively affect the way nutrients such as carbon and nitrogen are made available to plants and cycled in the soil.

Amazingly, 10-year average maize yields differed by less than 1% among the three systems, which were nearly equally profitable [154, 155]. The two organic systems showed increasing levels of available N, while N levels declined in the conventional system. This indicates that the organic systems are more sustainable, in terms of productivity, over the long term [141].

The soybean production systems were also highly productive, achieving 40 bushels/acre. In 1999, during one of the worst droughts on record, yields of organic soybeans were 30 bushels/acre, compared to only 16 bushels/acre from conventionally grown soybeans. Not only did organic practices encourage the soil to hold moisture more efficiently than conventionally managed soil, the higher organic-matter content also made organic soil less compact so that roots could penetrate more deeply to find moisture.

The results highlighted the benefits to soil quality organic farming brings, and its potential to avert crop failures. "Our trials show that improving the quality of the soil through organic practices can mean the difference between a harvest or hardship in times of drought", said Jeff Moyer, Farm Manager at Rodale Institute [156].

17

Cleaner Environment

Less Chemical Input, Less Leaching and Runoff

Sustainable agriculture systems that use little or no chemical pesticides or herbicides are clearly a benefit to the environment (see the next section). Moreover, conventional farming systems are often associated with problems such as nitrate leaching and groundwater pollution. Application of P fertilizers in excess of plant needs results in accumulation of available P in topsoils, and increased losses of surface water.

Water eutrophication is one of the starkest results of N and P pollution. The high nutrient concentrations stimulate algal blooms, which block sunlight, causing aquatic vegetation to die and, in the process, destroying valuable habitat, food and shelter for aquatic life. When the algae die and decompose, oxygen is used up, to the detriment of aquatic life.

Four farming systems—organic, low-input, conventional four-year rotation and conventional two-year rotation—were evaluated for tomatoes and corn from 1994 to 1998 in California's Sacramento Valley [157]. The organic and low-input systems showed 112% and 36% greater potentially mineralizable N pools than the conventional systems, respectively. However, as they used cover crops, there was a slower, more continuous release of mineral N throughout the growing season.

In contrast, conventional systems supplied mineral N in intervals from synthetic fertilizers, and N mineralization rates were 100% greater than in the organic and 28% greater than in the low-input system. This implied a greater likelihood of N leaching and creating associated pollution problems in conventional systems.

Average tomato and corn yields for the five-year period were not significantly different among the farming systems. The researchers concluded that the lower potential risk of N leaching from lower

N mineralization rates in the organic and low-input farming systems appear to improve agricultural sustainability and environmental quality while maintaining similar crop yields to conventional systems.

The 21-year Swiss study [149, 150] also assessed the extent to which organic farming practices would affect the accumulation of total and available P in soil, compared to conventional practices [158]. Soil samples were taken from a nonfertilized control, two conventionally cultivated treatments and two organically cultivated treatments.

Average annual P budgets of both organic farming systems were negative for each single rotation period and for the 21 years of field experimentation. This indicated that P removal by harvested products exceeded the P input by fertilizers. The conventionally cultivated soil, receiving mineral fertilizers and farmyard manure, showed a positive budget over all three rotations. Furthermore, the inorganic P availability in the topsoil decreased markedly in all treatments during the field trial except in the conventional treatment. Thus the potential for P pollution from organic systems was reduced.

The 15-year trials carried out by the Rodale Institute showed that the conventional system had greater environmental impacts— 60% more nitrate leached into groundwater over a five-year period than in the organic systems [154, 155]. Soils in the conventional system were also relatively high in water-soluble carbon, hence vulnerable to leaching out. The better water infiltration rates of the organic systems made them less prone to erosion and less likely to contribute to water pollution from surface runoff.

18

Reduced Pesticides and No Increase in Pests

Less Pesticides

Organic farming prohibits routine pesticide application. According to the Soil Association in the UK, about 430 synthetic pesticide-active ingredients are allowed in nonorganic farming, compared to seven in organic farming. The pesticides used in organic farming may only be used as the last resort for pest control when other methods fail. They are either natural or simple chemicals that degrade rapidly. Three of these require further authorization for use.

Many sustainable agriculture projects report large reductions in pesticide use after adopting integrated pest management. In Vietnam, farmers have cut the number of sprays from 3.4 to 1.0 per season, in Sri Lanka from 2.9 to 0.5 per season, and in Indonesia from 2.9 to 1.1 per season. Overall, in Southeast Asia, 100,000 small rice farmers involved in integrated pest management substantially increased yields while eliminating pesticides [130].

Pest Control Without Pesticides: No Crop Losses

Because organic procedures exclude synthetic pesticides, critics claim that losses due to pests would rise. However, research on California tomato production contradicted this claim [159]. There was no significant difference in levels of pest damage in 18 commercial farms, half of which were certified organic systems and half, conventional operations. Arthropod biodiversity was, on average, one-third greater in organic farms than in conventional farms. There was no significant difference between the two in herbivore (pest) abundance.

However, the natural enemies of pests were more abundant in organic farms, with greater species richness of all functional groups (herbivores, predators, parasitoids). Thus, any particular pest species in organic farms would be associated with a greater variety of herbivores (i.e., would be diluted) and subject to control by a wider variety and greater abundance of potential parasitoids and predators.

At the same time, research shows that pest control is achievable without pesticides, actually reversing crop losses. In East Africa, maize and sorghum face two major pests: stem borer and Striga, a parasitic plant. Field margins are planted with "trap crops" that attract stem borer, such as Napier grass and Sudan grass. Napier grass is a local weed whose odor attracts the stem borer. Pests are lured away from the crop into a trap—the grass produces a sticky substance that kills stem borer larvae [160]. The crops are interplanted with molasses grass (*Desmodium uncinatum*) and two legumes: silverleaf and greenleaf. The legumes bind N, enriching the soil. *Desmodium* also repels stem borers *and* Striga.

In Bangladesh, a project began in 1995 to promote nonchemical means of pest control in rice that relies on natural enemies and on the ability of the rice plant to compensate for insect damage. There have been no negative impacts on yields [161]. On the contrary, farmers using no insecticide consistently enjoy higher yields than those using insecticide. As project participants also modify other practices besides foregoing insecticides, it cannot be said that the yield increase is due entirely to the absence of insecticides. It does show, however, that insecticides are not needed to obtain yield increases. Project participants enjoy higher net returns than insecticide users: the 1998 average net return for participants was Tk 5373 ($107) per farmer per season compared to Tk 3443 ($69) for insecticide users.

Other Benefits of Avoiding Pesticides

Besides the obvious benefit of not using harmful pesticides, Korean researchers have reported that avoiding pesticides in paddy fields encourages the muddy loach fish, which effectively controls the mosquitoes that spread malaria and Japanese encephalitis [162]. Fields in which no insecticides were used had a richer variety of insect life. However, the fish are voracious predators of the mosquito larvae.

In Japan, an innovative organic farmer has pioneered a rice-growing system that turns weeds and pests into resources for raising ducks [163]. The ducks eat insect pests and the golden snail that attack rice plants, and also eat the seeds and seedlings of weeds. By using their feet to dig up the weed seedlings, the ducks aerate the water and provide mechanical stimulation to make the rice stalks strong and fertile. This practice has been adopted by about 10,000 farmers in Japan and by farmers in South Korea, Vietnam, the Philippines, Laos, Cambodia, Thailand and Malaysia. Many farmers increased their yield 20 to 50% or more in the first year. One farmer in Laos increased his income threefold.

Systems such as these, which are characteristic of sustainable agricultural approaches, make use of the complex interactions of different species, and show how important the relationship between biodiversity and agriculture is (see the next chapter).

The health benefits of avoiding pesticides are discussed briefly in "Organics for Health."

19

Supporting Biodiversity and Using Diversity

Agricultural Biodiversity Crucial for Food Security

Maintaining agricultural biodiversity is vital to long-term food security. Pimbert reviewed the multiple functions of agricultural biodiversity and its importance for rural livelihoods [164]. Agricultural biodiversity contributes to food and livelihood security, efficient production, environmental sustainability and rural development; it regenerates local food systems and rural economies. Rural people have dynamic and complex livelihoods, which usually rely on a diversity of plant and animal species, both wild and domesticated. Diversity *within* species (i.e., farmers' varieties or landraces) is also remarkable among the species domesticated for crop and livestock production, and results from rural people's innovation. Such agricultural diversity is vital insurance against crop and livestock disease outbreaks, and improves the long-term resilience of rural livelihoods to adverse trends or shocks. Agricultural biodiversity is increasingly threatened by the adoption of high-yielding, uniform cultivars and varieties in "modern" monoculture.

The proceedings of a 2002 FAO meeting on "Biodiversity and the Ecosystem Approach in Agriculture, Forestry and Fisheries" highlighted the interconnectedness of biodiversity and agriculture [165]. It gave specific examples of how farmers' innovations enhance biodiversity and the importance of biodiversity for agriculture. One paper reviewed 16 case studies from 10 countries in Asia, Latin America, Europe and Africa, showing how organic farming increases the diversity of genetic resources for food and agriculture [166]. In all cases, there is a close relationship between organic systems and the maintenance of biodiversity and improvement in the farmers' socioeconomic conditions.

Case studies of a community-based organic farming system in Bangladesh, the *ladang* cultivation of organic spices in Indonesia and organic coffee production in Mexico show how traditional and community-based management can rehabilitate abandoned and degraded agroecosystems. These polyculture systems are charac- terized by highly diversified ecosystems and agricultural biodiversity, which provide not only food, but also further community services. Case studies of organic cocoa farming in Mexico and organic, nat- urally pigmented cotton in Peru are examples of successful organic agriculture that have contributed to *in situ* conservation and sustain- able use in centers of diversity while providing economic benefits for local communities. Traditional and underutilized species and vari- eties in Peru (gluten-free quinoa), Italy (Saraceno grain, Zolfino bean, spelt wheat), and Indonesia (local varieties of rice) have been res- cued from extinction thanks to organic agriculture. Four case studies from Germany, Italy, South Africa and Brazil illustrate how organic farming has restored many traditional varieties and breeds that are better adapted to local ecological conditions and are resistant to disease. As the authors conclude, organic agriculture contributes to *in situ* conservation, restoration and maintenance of agricultural biodiversity.

Conserving and Supporting Biodiversity

Sustainable agriculture plays a further important role in conserving natural biodiversity. Organic farms often exhibit greater natural bio- diversity than conventional farms, with more trees, a wider diversity of crops and many different natural predators, which control pests and help prevent disease [131].

Research carried out in Colombia and Mexico found 90% fewer bird species in sun-grown coffee plantations as opposed to shade- grown organic coffee, which mimics the forests' natural habitat [167]. Shade cultivation is recommended by organic standards as it en- hances soil fertility, controls pests and diseases and expands crop production options. Another study by the British Trust for Ornithology found significantly higher breeding densities of skylark (an endan- gered species) on organic farms, compared to conventional farms. Floral diversity, which has also been threatened by the increasing use of herbicides in agricultural production, stands to benefit from organic systems that do not allow the use of chemical herbicides. Studies in Greece and England show that floral diversity and abun- dance is indeed higher in organic than in conventional systems.

Other studies show increased invertebrate diversity and abundance in organic systems.

A report from the Soil Association [168] comprehensively reviewed the findings of nine studies (seven from the UK, two from Denmark), and summarized the key findings of fourteen additional studies, on the biodiversity supported by organic farming. The report concluded that organic farming in the lowlands supports a much higher level of biodiversity (both abundance and diversity of species) than conventional farming systems, including species that have significantly declined. This was particularly true for wild plants in arable fields; birds and breeding skylarks; invertebrates, including arthropods that comprise bird food; nonpest butterflies; and spiders. Organic farms also showed significant decrease in pest aphids and no change in pest butterflies. Habitat quality was more favorable on organic farms, both in terms of field boundaries and crop habitats.

Many beneficial practices were identified with organic agriculture, such as crop rotations with grass leys (temporary pasture), mixed spring and autumn sowing, more permanent pasture, no application of herbicides or synthetic pesticides, and use of green manure. These practices can reverse the trends in the decline of biodiversity associated with conventional farming. Generally, the improvements in biodiversity were found across the cropped areas as well as at the field margins. The report also suggested that major benefits are likely in the uplands.

The reduced or nonuse of agrochemicals in organic and sustainable farming will also allow wild plant species to flourish, among which are an increasing number of herbs used in traditional medicines. The World Health Organization estimates that 75–80% of the world's population use plant medicines either in part or entirely for health care. Some of these wild plant species are facing extinction, and concerted effort is needed for their local conservation, while ensuring that harvesting from the wild is sustainable and continues to contribute to local people's livelihood [169]. Wild plants and animals are also part of an important repertoire of food and medicines for many farming communities [164].

Diversity Increases Agricultural Productivity

Biodiversity is an important and integral part of sustainable agricultural approaches. Each species in an agroecosystem is part of a web of ecological relationships connected by flows of energy and materials. In this sense, the different components of agrobiodiversity are multifunctional, and contribute to the resilience of production systems while providing environmental services, although some species may play key driving roles [164]. The environmental services provided by agricultural biodiversity include soil organic-matter decomposition, nutrient cycling, biomass production and yield efficiency, soil and water conservation, pest control, pollination and dispersal, biodiversity conservation, climate functions, water cycling and influence on landscape structure.

Empirical evidence from a study conducted since 1994 shows that biodiverse ecosystems are two to three times more productive than monocultures [170, 171]. In experimental plots, both aboveground and total biomass increased significantly with species number. The high-diversity plots were fairly immune to the invasion and growth of weeds, but this was not so for monocultures and low-diversity plots. Thus, biodiverse systems are more productive, and less prone to weeds as well!

Proving with stunning results that planting a diversity of crops is beneficial (compared with monocultures), thousands of Chinese rice farmers have doubled yields and nearly eliminated its most devastating disease without using chemicals or spending more [172, 173]. Scientists worked together with farmers in Yunnan, who implemented a simple practice that radically restricted the rice blast fungus that destroys millions of tons of rice and costs farmers several billion dollars in losses each year.

Instead of planting large stands of a single type of rice, as is typical, farmers planted a mixture of two varieties: a standard hybrid rice that does not usually succumb to rice blast and a much more valuable glutinous or "sticky" rice known to be very susceptible. The genetically diverse rice crops were planted in all the rice fields in five townships in 1998 (812 hectares) and ten townships in 1999 (3342 hectares).

Disease-susceptible varieties planted with resistant varieties had 89% greater yield, and blast was 94% less severe than when grown in monoculture. Both glutinous and hybrid rice showed decreased infection. The hypothesis is fairly clear for glutinous rice. If a variety is susceptible to a disease, the more concentrated those susceptible types are, the more easily disease spreads. It is less likely to spread when susceptible plants are grown among plants resistant to the disease (i.e., a dilution effect occurs). The glutinous rice plants, which rise above the shorter hybrid rice, also enjoyed sunnier, warmer and drier conditions that discouraged fungal growth. Disease reduction in the hybrid variety may be due to the taller glutinous rice blocking the airborne spores of rice blast, and to greater induced resistance (due to diverse fields supporting diverse pathogens with no single dominant strain). The gross value per hectare of the mixtures was 14% greater than hybrid monocultures and 40% greater than glutinous monocultures.

In Cuba, integrated farming systems or polycultures, such as cassava-beans-maize, cassava-tomato-maize, and sweet potato-maize have 1.45 to 2.82 times greater productivity than monocultures [135]. In addition, legumes improve the physical and chemical characteristics of soil and effectively break the cycle of insect-pest infestations.

Integrating vegetables into rice-farming systems in Bangladesh by planting them on dikes has not affected rice yields, despite the area lost to dike crops [161]. Instead, the vegetables provided families with more nutrients. The surplus was shared with neighbors, friends and relatives, or sold, providing an added value of 14%.

Integrating fish into flooded rice systems also caused no significant decline in rice yields and in some cases increased yields. Net returns from selling the fish averaged Tk 7354 ($147) per farmer per season, more than the returns from rice. As with vegetables, rice–fish farmers ate fish more frequently and donated much of it to their social networks.

Soil biodiversity also plays a crucial role in promoting sustainable and productive agriculture, and organic practices help enhance this [174]. Organic mulch, applied judiciously to degraded and crusted soil surfaces in the Sahelian region of Burkina Faso, triggered termite activity, promoting the recovery and rehabilitation of degraded soils. Termites feeding on or transporting surface-applied mulch improved soil structure and water infiltration, enhancing nutrient release into the soil. The growth and yield of cowpeas were far better on plots with termites than on plots without. In India, organic fertilizers and vermicultured earthworms applied in trenches between tea rows increased tea yields by 76–239%, compared to conventional inorganic fertilization. Profits increased accordingly.

20

Environmental and Economic Sustainability

Sustainable Production

Research published in *Nature* investigated the sustainability of organic, conventional and integrated (combining both methods) apple production systems in Washington from 1994–1999 [175, 176]. The organic system ranked first in terms of environmental and economic sustainability, the integrated system, second, and the conventional system was ranked last. The indicators used were soil quality, horticultural performance, orchard profitability, environmental quality and energy efficiency.

Soil quality ratings in 1998 and 1999 for the organic and integrated systems were significantly higher than for the conventional system, due to the addition of compost and mulch. All three systems gave comparable yields, with no observable differences in physiological disorders or pest and disease damage. There were satisfactory levels of nutrients for all. A consumer taste test found organic apples less tart at harvest and sweeter than conventional apples after the apples were stored for six months.

Organic apples were the most profitable due to price premiums and quicker investment return. Despite initial lower receipts in the first three years, due to the time taken to convert to certified organic farming, the price premium in the next three years averaged 50% above conventional prices. In the long term, the organic system recovered costs faster. The study projected that the organic system would break even after 9 years, but that the conventional system would do so only after 15 years, and the integrated system, after 17 years.

Environmental impact was assessed by a rating index to determine potential adverse impacts of pesticides and fruit thinners: the higher the rating, the greater the negative impact. The rating of the conventional system was 6.2 times that of the organic system. Despite higher labor needs, the organic system expended less energy on fertilizer, weed control and biological control of pests, making it the most energy efficient.

Another study evaluated the financial and environmental aspects of sustainability of organic, integrated and conventional farming systems by applying an integrated economic-environmental accounting framework to three farms in Tuscany, Italy [177]. In terms of financial performance, the gross margins of steady-state organic farming systems were higher than the corresponding conventional farming systems' gross margins. The organic systems performed better than the integrated and conventional systems with respect to nitrogen losses, pesticide risk, herbaceous plant biodiversity and most other environmental indicators. The results provided evidence that organic farming potentially improves the efficiency of many environmental indicators, and it is remunerative. While not fully conclusive that organic farming is more sustainable; nonetheless, the performance of organic farming systems was better than that of conventional farming systems.

Environmentally Sustainable

A Europe-wide study assessed environmental and resource use impacts of organic farming, relative to conventional farming [178]. The study showed that organic farming performs better than conventional farming in relation to the majority of environmental indicators reviewed. In no category did organic farming show a worse performance when compared with conventional farming.

For example, organic farming performed better than conventional farming in terms of floral and faunal diversity, wildlife conservation and habitat diversity. Organic farming also conserved soil fertility and system stability better than conventional systems. Furthermore, the study showed that organic farming results in lower or similar nitrate leaching rates than integrated or conventional agriculture, and that it does not pose any risk of ground and surface water pollution from synthetic pesticides.

The FAO review [133] concluded, "As a final assessment, it can be stated that well-managed organic agriculture leads to more favorable conditions at *all* environmental levels" (italics added, p.62).

Its assessment showed that organic-matter content is usually higher in organic soils, indicating higher fertility, stability and moisture-retention capacity, which reduce the risk of erosion and desertification.

Organic soils have significantly higher biological activity and a higher mass of microorganisms, making for more rapid nutrient recycling and improved soil structure.

The review found that organic agriculture poses no risk of water pollution through synthetic pesticides and that nitrate leaching rates per hectare are significantly lower compared to conventional systems. In terms of energy use, organic agriculture performs better than conventional agriculture (see next section).

The review established that genetic resources, including insects and microorganisms, all increase when land is farmed organically, while wild flora and fauna within and around organic farms are more diverse and abundant. By offering food resources and shelter for beneficial arthropods and birds, organic agriculture contributes to natural pest control. It also contributes to the conservation and survival of pollinators.

21

Ameliorating Climate Change

Energy Efficiency

"Modern" agriculture has a lot to answer for in terms of contributing to climate change, which is by far the most daunting problem that humans have ever encountered. It has increased emissions of nitrous oxide and methane, potent greenhouse gases; it is fossil-fuel energy intensive and thus contributes to the loss of soil carbon to the atmosphere [179].

Sustainable agricultural practices can provide synergistic benefit toward ameliorating climate change. The FAO believes that organic agriculture enables ecosystems to better adjust to the effects of climate change and has major potential for reducing agricultural greenhouse gas emissions [133]. Its review concluded that "Organic agriculture performs better than conventional agriculture on a per hectare scale, both with respect to direct energy consumption (fuel and oil) and indirect consumption (synthetic fertilizers and pesticides)," with high efficiency of energy use (p.61).

The Rodale Institute's trials found that energy use in the conventional system was 200% higher than in either of the organic systems [141]. Research in Finland showed that while organic farming used more machine hours than conventional farming, total energy consumption was still lowest in organic systems [180]. In conventional systems, more than half of total energy consumed in rye production was spent on the manufacture of pesticides.

Organic agriculture was more energy efficient than conventional agriculture in apple production systems [175, 176]. Studies in Denmark compared organic and conventional farming for milk and barley grain production [181]. The total energy used per kilogram of milk produced was lower in the organic than in the conventional dairy farm, while the total energy used to grow a hectare of organic spring barley was 35% lower than used to produce conventional spring barley on the same area. However, organic yield was lower, thus energy used to produce one kg of barley was only marginally lower for the organic than for the conventional.

Carbon dioxide (CO_2) emissions were calculated to be 48–66% lower per hectare in organic farming systems in Europe [133, 178], and were attributed to the characteristics of organic agriculture [i.e., no input of mineral N fertilizers with high energy consumption, lower use of high-energy-consuming feedstuffs, lower input of mineral fertilizers (P, K) and elimination of pesticides].

Furthermore, because of sustainable agriculture's focus on local production, consumption and distribution, less energy is wasted on transportation of products, particularly by air. According to a study carried out in 2001, greenhouse gas emissions associated with the transport of food from a local farm to a farmer's market were 650 times lower than emissions associated with the average food sold in supermarkets [cited in 179].

Greater Carbon Sequestration

Soils are an important sink for atmospheric CO_2, but this sink has been increasingly depleted by conventional agricultural land use. Sustainable agriculture approaches, however, help to counteract climate change by restoring soil organic-matter content (see "Better Soils"), as these increase carbon fixation below ground. Organic matter is restored by the addition of manures, compost, mulches and cover crops.

Pretty and Hine suggest that the 208 projects they assessed accumulated some 55.1 million tons of carbon (C) [130]. The SAFS Project found that organic C content of the soil increased in both organic and low-input systems [143], while the study of 20 commercial farms in California found that organic fields had 28% more organic C [148].

This was also true in the 15-year study by the Rodale Institute, where soil C levels increased in the two organic systems, but not in the conventional system [141]. The researchers concluded that organic systems showed significant ability to absorb and retain C, raising the possibility that sustainable agriculture practices can help reduce the impact of global warming.

Less Nitrous Oxide Emissions

The FAO also estimated that organic agriculture is likely to emit less nitrous oxide (N_2O) [133], another important greenhouse gas and also a cause of stratospheric ozone depletion. This is due to lower N inputs; less N from organic manure due to lower livestock densities; higher C/N ratios of applied organic manure and less available mineral N in the soil as a source of denitrification; and efficient uptake of mobile N in soils due to cover crops.

22

Efficient and Profitable Production

Productivity Enhanced

Any yield decrease in organic agriculture is more than made up for by its ecological and efficiency gains and lower costs, making it a profitable venture. The Swiss study found that input of fertilizer and energy was reduced by 34–53% and pesticide input by 97%, whereas mean crop yield was only 20% lower over the 21 years, indicating efficient production and resource use [149, 150]. The organic approach was commercially viable in the long term, producing more food per unit of energy or resources.

Data show that smaller farms produce far more per unit area than larger farms (which tend to be monocultures characteristic of conventional farming) [136]. Though the yield per unit area of one crop may be lower on a small farm than on a large monoculture, the total output per unit area, often composed of more than a dozen crops and various animal products, can be far higher. Small farms are also more efficient than large ones in terms of land use and "total factor productivity," an averaging of the efficiency of use of all the different factors that go into production, including land, labor, inputs and capital.

Studies in Bolivia show that though yields are greater in chemically fertilized and machinery-prepared potato fields, energy costs are higher and net economic benefits lower, than where native legumes have been used as rotational crops [135]. Surveys indicate that farmers prefer the latter alternative system because it optimizes the use of scarce resources, labor and available capital, and is accessible to even poor producers.

Lower Costs, Higher Profits

Two trials in Minnesota evaluated a two-year corn-soybean rotation and a four-year corn-soybean-oat/alfalfa-alfalfa crop rotation under four management strategies: zero, low, high and organic inputs [182]. Averaged across a seven-year time frame from 1993–1999, corn and soybean yields in the four-year organic strategy were 91 and 93%, and 81 and 84%, respectively, of the two-year high-input strategy. However, oat yields were similar with either the four-year organic or high-input strategies. Alfalfa yields in the four-year organic strategy were 92% that of the four-year high-input strategy in one trial, and in the second trial, yields were the same.

Despite the slight reduction in corn and soybean yields, the organic systems had lower production costs than the high-input strategy. Consequently, net returns, without considering organic price premiums, for the two strategies were equivalent. The scientists suggested that organic production systems could be competitive with conventional ones.

A comprehensive review of the many comparison studies of grain and soybean production conducted by six U.S. Midwestern universities since 1978 found that, in general, organic production was equivalent to, and in some cases better than, conventional means [183]. Organic systems had higher yields than conventional systems that featured continuous crop production (i.e., no crop rotations), and equal or lower yields than conventional systems that included crop rotations. In drier climates, organic systems had higher yields, as they were more drought-hardy than conventional systems.

The organic cropping systems were always more profitable than the most common conventional systems if organic price premiums were factored in. When the higher premiums were not factored in, the organic systems were still more productive and profitable in half the studies. This was attributed to lower production costs and the ability of organic systems to outperform the conventional systems in drier areas, or during drier periods. The author concluded, "organic production systems are competitive with the most common conventional production systems," and suggested that, "if farmers obtain current market premiums for organic grains and soybeans, their organic production generally delivers higher profits than nonorganic grain and soybean production" (p.2).

The 15-year results from the Rodale Institute showed that after a transition period with lower yields, the organic systems were competitive financially with the conventional systems [141]. While the costs of the transition are likely to affect a farm's overall financial picture for some years, projected profits ranged from slightly below to substantially above those of the conventional system, even though economic analyses did not assume any organic price premium. The higher profits for the organic farms came largely from higher corn yields, which nearly doubled after the transition period. When prices or yields were low, organic farms suffered less than the conventional and had fewer income fluctuations, as they had a diversity of crops other than corn to sell. Expenses on the organic farms were significantly lower than on the conventional farms—the latter spent 95% more on fertilizers and pesticides. Overall production costs on the organic farms were 26% lower.

23

Improved Food Security and Benefits to Local Communities

Increased Local Food Production

Despite adequate global food production, many still go hungry because increased food supply does not automatically mean increased food security. What is important is who produces the food, who has access to the technology and knowledge to produce it, and who has the purchasing power to acquire it [130]. Poor farmers cannot afford expensive "modern" technologies that theoretically raise yields.

Many farmers show "lagging productivity," not because they lack "miracle" seeds that contain their own insecticide or tolerate massive doses of herbicide, but because they have been displaced onto marginal, rain-fed lands, and face structures and macroeconomic policies that have built on historical inequalities and that are increasingly inimical to food production by small farmers [184].

As such, their agriculture is best characterized as "complex, diverse and risk-prone" [185], and they have tailored agricultural technologies to their variable but unique circumstances in terms of local climate, topography, soils, biodiversity, cropping systems, resources, and other elements. It is these farmers, already risk-prone, who stand to be harmed most by the risks of GM crops [184].

Sustainable agricultural approaches must thus allow farmers to improve local food production with low-cost, readily available technologies and inputs, without causing environmental damage. This was indeed the case, as reviewed by Pretty and Hine [130]. Most sustainable agriculture projects and initiatives reported significant increases in household food production—some as yield improvements, some as increases in cropping intensity or diversity of produce.

The evidence showed:

- Average food production per household increased by 1.71 tons per year (up 73%) for 4.42 million farmers on 3.58 million hectares.
- Increase in food production was 17 tons per year (an increase of 150%) for 146,000 farmers on 542,000 hectares cultivating roots (potato, sweet potato and cassava).
- Total production increased by 150 tons per household (an increase of 46%) for the larger farms in Latin America (average size 90 hectares).

The review found that as food supply increased, domestic consumption also increased, with direct health benefits, particularly for women and children. Furthermore, 88% of the 208 projects made better use of locally available natural resources, and 92% improved human capital through learning programs. In more than half the projects, people worked together.

Learning from Farmers

Sustainable agricultural approaches recognize the value of traditional and indigenous knowledge, and of farmers' experience and innovation. The importance and value of learning from farmers, and of farmer-led participatory agricultural research, are well established in concepts such as "farmer first" [185, 186].

Case studies and experiences of successful agroecological innovations from Africa, Latin America and Asia [187] provide evidence that low-external-input agriculture using agroecological practices could make an important contribution to feeding the world over the next 30 to 50 years. Relying on mainly local resources and knowledge, farmers are able to increase yields substantially, sometimes doubling or tripling outputs.

To cite one example, in Mali's Sahelian Zone, soil and water conservation practices and agroforestry have increased cereal yields, in some cases from 300 kg/ha to 1700 kg/ha, about twice the level needed to meet basic food needs. Emphasis has also been placed on conserving traditional varieties of seeds and biodiversity, through farmer-based evaluation and community or local gene banks.

The FAO review highlights the important contributions of resource-poor farmers worldwide [133]. Noncertified organic agriculture, practiced by millions of indigenous people, peasants and small family farms make a significant contribution to regional food security: in Latin America they account for more than 50% of the maize, beans, manioc and potatoes produced; in Africa, most of the cereals, roots and tubers; in Asia, most of the rice.

Case studies from India, Brazil, Iran, Thailand and Uganda show how traditional knowledge, innovation and agroecological approaches have brought numerous benefits: increased productivity, better environmental health and soil fertility, improved biodiversity, economic benefits, food security, enhanced social relations within communities and revival of traditional, sustainable agricultural practices [133].

Farmers in Ethiopia are taking steps to ensure their food security by relying on their knowledge [188]. In Ejere, farmers have reclaimed their own varieties of local wheat, *teff* (an Ethiopian staple cereal) and barley, after so-called "modern high-yielding varieties" actually resulted in lower yields and other problems. In the Butajira area, farmers are demonstrating that it is possible to farm intensively and sustainably to provide enough food to meet population needs. They do this by using indigenous crops selected for resistance to diseases, drought tolerance and many other desirable features, by intercropping and by integrating livestock management. In Worabe, farmers are maintaining a complex, sustainable and indigenous agricultural system that ensures food security. The system is based on *enset*, a very drought-resistant, multiple-use, indigenous crop.

Better Incomes, Increased Food Security

Evidence from hundreds of grassroots development projects shows that increasing agricultural productivity with agroecological practices not only increases food supplies, but also increases incomes, thus reducing poverty, increasing food access, reducing malnutrition and improving the livelihoods of the poor [189]. Agroecological systems lead to more stable levels of total production per unit area than high-input systems; they give more economically favorable rates of return, provide a return to labor and other inputs for a livelihood acceptable to small farmers and their families. They also ensure soil protection and conservation and enhance agrobiodiversity [190].

Integrated production systems and diversified farms have helped farmers in south-central Chile reach year-round food self-sufficiency while rebuilding the land's productive capacity [135]. Small, model farm systems have been set up, consisting of polycultures and rotating sequences of forage and food crops, forest and fruit trees, and incorporating livestock.

Soil fertility improved, and no serious pest or disease problems have appeared. Fruit trees and forage crops achieved higher than average yields, and milk and egg production far exceeded that on conventional high-input farms. For a typical family, such systems produced a 250% surplus of protein, 80% and 550% surpluses of vitamin A and C, respectively, and a 330% surplus of calcium. If all the farm output were sold at wholesale prices, a family could generate a monthly net income 1.5 times greater than the monthly minimum wage in Chile, while dedicating only a few hours per week to the farm. The time freed up could be used for other income-generating activities.

Organic agriculture could improve income, profitability and return on labor by removing or reducing the need for purchased inputs; by diversification (often adding a new productive element) and optimizing productivity; by maintaining or improving on- and off-farm biodiversity, allowing farmers to market noncultivated crops, insects and animals; and by sales in a premium market [191]. A case study from Senegal showed that yields could be increased manifold, and were less variable year to year, with consequent improvements in household food security. Likewise, a participatory fair-trade coffee cooperative in Mexico, which adopted organic practices, allowed smallholder coffee growers to overcome soil degradation and low yields, and to gain access to a speciality market.

Generating Money for the Local Economy

Money flows of an organic box scheme from Cusgarne Organics (UK) showed the benefit to the community at large of buying locally [192]. The economic analysis followed the trail of the farm box-scheme income, monitoring exactly where the money was spent, how much of it was "local" expenditure, and then tracked that money to the next layer of spending.

It estimated that for every £1 spent at Cusgarne Organics, £2.59 is generated for the local economy. In contrast, a study involving supermarket giants Asda and Tesco found that for every £1 spent at a supermarket, only £1.40 is generated for the local economy. The study concludes: "The figures demonstrate that the net effect of spending at Cusgarne Organics to the local economy is nearly double the effect of the same amount spent with out-of-county and national businesses" (p. 16).

24

Organics for Health

Less Chemical Residues

A comprehensive Soil Association review of scientific research has shown that, on average, organic food is better than nonorganic food [193]. First, it is safer, as organic farming prohibits routine pesticide and herbicide use, so chemical residues are rarely found. In contrast, nonorganic food is likely to be contaminated with residues that often occur in potentially dangerous combinations. The British Society for Allergy, Environmental and Nutritional Medicine, commenting on the report, states: "We have long believed the micronutrient deficiencies common in our patients have their roots in the mineral-depletion of soils by intensive agriculture, and *suspect that pesticide exposures are contributing to the alarming rise in allergies and other illnesses*" (italics added).

The negative effects of pesticides on health include neurotoxicity, disruption of the endocrine system, carcinogenicity and immune system suppression (see also "Herbicide Hazards"). The impacts of dietary exposure to pesticide residues at levels typically found in and on food are less easy to establish, but a precautionary approach is necessary. While there are recommended safety levels for pesticides, the British government's own tests have shown that average residue levels on foods may be underreported.

Research has also suggested that pesticide exposure affects male reproductive function, resulting in decreased fertilizing ability of the sperm and reduced fertilization rates [194]. Correspondingly, members of a Danish organic farmers' association, whose intake of organic dairy products was at least 50% of total intake of dairy products, had high sperm density [195]. In another study, sperm concentration was 43.1% higher among men eating organically produced food [196].

Children, in particular, may stand to benefit from organic food. Scientists monitored preschool children in Seattle, Washington to assess their exposure to organophosphorus (OP) pesticide from diet [197]. The total dimethyl metabolite concentration was approximately six times higher for children with conventional diets than those with organic diets. The calculated dose estimates suggest that consumption of organic fruits, vegetables and juice can reduce children's exposure levels from above to below the U.S. Environmental Protection Agency's guidelines, thereby shifting exposures from a range of uncertain risk to a range of negligible risk. The study concluded that consumption of organic produce could be a relatively simple way for parents to reduce children's exposure to OP pesticides.

Healthier and More Nutritious

Additionally, organic food production bans the use of artificial food additives (hydrogenated fats, phosphoric acid, aspartame and monosodium glutamate), which have been linked to health problems as diverse as heart disease, osteoporosis, migraines and hyperactivity [193].

Furthermore, while plants extract a wide range of minerals from the soil, artificial fertilizers replace only a few principal minerals. There is a clear long-term decline in the trace-mineral content of fruit and vegetables, and the influence of farming practices needs to be investigated more thoroughly. The Soil Association review [193] found that, on average, organic food has higher vitamin C, higher mineral levels and higher phytonutrients—plant compounds that can fight cancer (see later)—than conventional food.

Conventional produce also tends to contain more water than organic produce, which contains more dry matter (on average, 20% more) for a given total weight [193]. Thus, the higher cost of fresh organic produce is partly offset by purchasers of conventional produce paying for the extra weight of water and getting only 83% of the nutrients, on average, available in organic produce. The higher water content also tends to dilute nutrient content.

Tests with people and animals eating organic food show it makes a real difference to health, and alternative cancer therapies have achieved good results relying on the exclusive consumption of organic food. The review [193] cites recent clinical evidence from doctors and nutritionists administering alternative cancer treatments, who have observed that a completely organic diet is essential for a successful outcome. Nutritional cancer therapies avoid pollutants and toxins as much as possible and promote exclusive consumption of organically grown foods and increases in nutrient intakes. Animal feeding trials have also demonstrated better reproductive health, better growth, and better recovery from illness.

A literature review of 41 studies and 1240 comparisons [198] found statistically significant differences in the nutrient content of organic and conventional crops. This was attributed primarily to differences in soil fertility management and its effects on soil ecology and plant metabolism. Organic crops contained significantly more nutrients—vitamin C, iron, magnesium and phosphorus—and significantly less nitrates (a toxic compound) than conventional crops. There were nonsignificant trends showing less protein in organic crops. However, organic crops were of a better quality and had higher content of nutritionally significant minerals, with lower amounts of some heavy metals compared to conventional ones.

Helping Fight Cancer

Plant phenolics (flavonoids) are plant secondary metabolites thought to protect plants against insect predation, bacterial and fungal infection and photo-oxidation. These plant chemicals have been found to be effective in preventing cancer and heart disease, and to combat age-related neurological dysfunctions. A recent scientific paper [199, 200] compared the total phenolic (TP) content of marionberries, strawberries and corn grown by organic and other sustainable methods with conventional agricultural practices. Statistically higher levels of TPs were consistently found in organically and sustainably grown foods as compared to those produced by conventional agriculture.

An earlier study comparing antioxidant compounds in organic and conventional peaches and pears established that an improvement in the antioxidant defence system of the plants occurred as a consequence of organic cultivation practices [201]. This is likely to exert protection against fruit damage when grown in the absence of pesticides. Hence organic agriculture, which eliminates the routine use of synthetic pesticides and chemical fertilizers, could create conditions favorable to the production of health-enhancing plant phenolics.

These and many other health benefits of organic foods have been brought to the attention of the British government [202, 203]. Among the issues raised are the hidden costs of conventional agriculture, which are not factored into the price. If hidden costs were taken into account, conventionally produced food would prove more expensive than organic food. For example, avoidance of the BSE ("mad cow disease") epidemic through organic farming would have saved £4.5 billion. No animal born and raised on an organic farm developed BSE in Great Britain.

25

Conclusion to Part 3

Sustainable agricultural approaches can deliver substantial increases in food production at low cost. They can be economically, environmentally and socially viable, and contribute positively to local livelihoods. They are also better for health and the environment.

Because the true root cause of hunger is inequality among nations and peoples, any method of boosting food production that deepens inequality is bound to fail to reduce hunger. Conversely, only technologies that have positive effects on the distribution of wealth, income and assets can truly reduce hunger [4]. Fortunately, such technologies already exist in sustainable approaches to agriculture.

Agroecology, sustainable agriculture and organic farming work, not just for farmers in the developed world, but especially for farmers in developing countries. As the FAO review [133] shows, there is a good existing base to build and scale up efforts for both certified and noncertified organic agriculture. The technologies and social processes for local improvements are increasingly well tested and established, and already delivering benefits in terms of increased productivity. The examples reviewed here are only a foretaste of the myriad successful experiences of sustainable agricultural practices at the local level. They represent countless demonstrations of talent, creativity and scientific capability in rural communities [132].

There is thus an urgent need to concentrate effort, research, funds and policy support on agroecology, sustainable agriculture and organic farming, particularly strengthening production by farmers themselves for local needs. The challenge is to scale up and multiply the successes, as well as to make them equitably and broadly accessible. The model of "modern" agriculture, so often in the hands of a few large corporations, must be challenged, as must be GM crops. Existing subsidies and policy incentives for conventional chemical and GM approaches need to be dismantled, and brakes applied on the drain of resources away from the alternatives [4]. We also need to guard against organic agriculture being taken over by powerful interests, and support all kinds of sustainable agriculture, especially that on small farms.

References

1. "Open Letter from World Scientists to All Governments" calling for a moratorium on releases of GMOs and support for organic sustainable agriculture, now signed by more than 600 scientists from 72 countries, with many references to the scientific literature (www.i-sis.org.uk).

2. *Agriculture: Towards 2015/30.* FAO Global Perspectives Studies Unit, July 2000.

3. Altieri, M. A. and Rosset, P. Ten reasons why biotechnology will not ensure food security, protect the environment and reduce poverty in the developing world. *AgBioForum*, Volume 2, Number 3 & 4, Summer/Fall 1999, 155–162.

4. Altieri, M. A. and Rosset, P. Strengthening the case for why biotechnology will not help the developing world: A response to McGloughlin. *AgBioForum*, Volume 2, Number 3 & 4, Summer/Fall 1999, 226–236.

5. ActionAid. *GM Crops—Going Against the Grain*, 2003 (http://www.actionaid.org/resources/pdfs/gatg.pdf).

6. http://www.isaaa.org/

7. Pimbert, M., Wakeford, T., and Satheesh, P. V. Citizens' juries on GMOs and farming futures in India. *LEISA Magazine*, December 2001, 27–30 (http://www.ileia.org/2/17-4/27-30.PDF).

8. Pimbert, M. P. and Wakeford, T. *Prajateerpu: A Citizens Jury/Scenario Workshop on Food and Farming Futures for Andhra Pradesh, India.* IIED & IDS, 2002 (http://www.iied.org/pdf/Prajateerpu.pdf).

9. Ho, M. W. and Lim, L. C. Biotech debacle in four parts. Special briefing for the Prime Minister's Strategy Unit on GM. *ISIS Report*, August 2002 (www.i-sis.org.uk).

10. Ho, M. W. The state of the art. The continuing debacle of an industry both financially and scientifically bankrupt. *GeneWatch* (in press), 2003.

11. "Monsanto investors face catastrophic risk," Greenpeace, Berlin, Press Release, 16 April, 2003.

12. Benbrook, C. M. Evidence of the magnitude and consequences of the Roundup Ready soybean yield drag from university-based varietal trials in 1998. *AgBioTech InfoNet Technical Paper Number 1*, 1999; Troubled times

amid commercial success: Glyphosate efficacy in slipping and unstable transgenic expression erodes plant defences and yields. *AgBioTech InfoNet Technical Paper Number 4*, 1999 (www.biotech-infonet/RR_yield_less.html).

13. Benbrook, C. Do GM crops mean less pesticide use? *Pesticide Outlook*, October 2001.

14. Lim, L. C. and Matthews, J. 2002. GM crops failed on every count. *Science in Society* 13/14:31–33; fully referenced version on ISIS members' Web site, www.i-sis.org.uk.

15. *Seeds of doubt, North American farmers' experiences of GM crops.* Soil Association, 2002, ISBN 0-905200-89-6.

16. Shiva, V. and Jafri, A. H. Failure of the GMOs in India. *Research Foundation for Science, Technology and Ecology Report*, 2003; see also Ho, M. W. *Living with the Fluid Genome.* ISIS & TWN, London and Penang, 2003. Chapter 1, p. 39.

17. Finnegan, H. and McElroy, D. 1994. Transgene inactivation: plants fight back! *Bio/Technology* 12:883–888.

18. Ho, M. W. *Living with the Fluid Genome.* ISIS & TWN, London and Penang, 2003. Chapter 11, Section, "Transgenic instability, the best kept open secret."

19. Ho, M.W., Cummins, J. and Ryan, A. *ISIS Reprints on Transgenic Instability 1999–2002*, ISIS members' Web site, www.i-sis.org.uk.

20. Gahakwa, D., Maqbool, S. B., Fu, X., Sudhakar, D., Christou, P. and Kohli, A. 2000. Transgenic rice as a system to study the stability of transgene expression: multiple heterologous transgenes show similar behavior in diverse genetic backgrounds. *Theor. Appl. Genet.* 101:388–399.

21. Ho, M. W. Questionable stability at JIC. *ISIS News* 9/10, July 2001. ISSN: 1474–1547 (print), ISSN: 1474–1814 (online), www.i-sis.org.uk, reviewing ref. 20.

22. Hall, L., Topinka, K., Huffman, J., Davis, L. and Good, A. 2000. Pollen flow between herbicide-resistant *Brassica napus* is the cause of multiple-resistant *B. napus* volunteers. *Weed Science*, 48:688–694.

23. Orson, J. Gene stacking in herbicide tolerant oilseed rape: lessons from the North American experience. "English Nature Research Reports No. 443." *English Nature*, Jan. 2002, ISSN 0967-876X.

24. Ho, M. W. and Cummins, J. 2002. What's wrong with GMOs? *Science in Society* 16:11–27; fully referenced version on ISIS members' Web site, www.i-sis.org.uk.

25. Cummins, J. and Ho, M. W. 2003. Atrazine poisoning worse than suspected. *Science in Society* 17:22–23; fully referenced version on ISIS members' Web site, www.i-sis.org.uk.

26. "Engineered Genes Help Wild Weeds Thrive" by Cat Lazaroff, *Environmental News Service*, Washington, USA, 9 August 2002.

27. Lim, L. C. Environmental and Health Impacts of Bt crops. *ISIS Report,* April, 2003; containing 63 references.

28. Quist, D. and Chapela, I. H. 2001. Transgenic DNA introgressed into traditional maize landraces in Oaxaca, Mexico. *Nature* 414:541–543.

29. Ho, M. W. and Cummins, J. 2002. Who's afraid of horizontal gene transfer? *ISIS Report,* 4 March 2002 (www.i-sis.org.uk); also The GM maize war in three episodes. *Science in Society* 15:12–14.

30. Ho, M. W. 2002. Worst ever contamination of Mexican landraces. *ISIS Report,* 29 April 2002 (www.i-sis.org.uk); also The GM maize war in three episodes. *Science in Society* 15:12–14.

31. Ho, M.W. 2002. Canadian farmers against corporate serfdom. *Science in Society* 16:5–6.

32. Kietke, L. Research shows: herbicide tolerance everywhere. *Manitoba Co-operator,* August 1, 2002; Friesen, L. F., Nelson, A. F. and Van Acker, R. C. Evidence of contamination of pedigreed canola (*Brassica napus*) seedlots in Western Canada with genetically engineered herbicide resistance traits. *Agronomy Journal* (in press).

33. *GM Crops: What you should know, A guide to both the science and implications of commercialisation of genetically modified crops,* GM Free Cymru, June 2002 (www.gm-news.co.uk).

34. Meier, P. and Wackernagel, W. 2003. Monitoring the spread of recombinant DNA from field plots with transgenic sugar beet plants by PCR and natural transformation of *Pseudomonas stutzeri. Transgenic Research* 12:293–304.

35. Saunders, P. T. Use and abuse of the precautionary principle. *ISIS News* 6, September 2000, ISSN: 1474–1547 (print), ISSN: 1474–1814 (online), www.i-sis.org.uk.

36. Saunders, P. T. and Ho, M. W. The precautionary principle and scientific evidence. *ISIS News* 7/8, February 2001, ISSN: 1474–1547 (print), ISSN: 1474–1814 (online), www.i-sis.org.uk; also *TWN Biosafety Briefing Paper,* December 2002.

37. Saunders, P. T. and Ho, M. W. The precautionary principle is science-based. *ISIS Report,* April 2003 (www.i-sis.org.uk).

38. Ho, M. W. FAQs on genetic engineering. *ISIS Tutorials* (www.i-sis.org.uk); also *TWN Biosafety Briefing Paper,* December 2002.

39. Ho, M. W. and Steinbrecher, R. 1998. Fatal flaws in food safety assessment: Critique of the joint FAO/WHO Biotechnology and Food Safety Report. *Journal of Nutritional and Environmental Interactions* 2:1–84.

40. Conner, A. J. 1995. Case study: food safety evaluation of transgenic potato. In *Application of the Principle of Substantial Equivalence to the Safety Evaluation of Foods or Food Components from Plants Derived by Modern Biotechnology,* pp. 23–35, WHO/FNU/FOS/95.1. World Health Organization, Geneva, Switzerland.

REFERENCES

41. Martineau, B. *First Fruit*. McGraw-Hill, New York, 2001.

42. *Greenpeace Business*, Issue 66, April/May 2002.

43. *Late lessons from early warnings: The precautionary principle 1896–2000.* Edited by: Poul Harremoës, David Gee, Malcolm MacGarvin, Andy Stirling, Jane Keys, Brian Wynne, Sofia Guedes Vaz. Environmental issue report No 22, 2002, OPOCE (Office for Official Publications of the European Communities).

44. Response by Stanley William Barclay Ewen, M.B.Ch.B., Ph.D., F.R.C. Path to Health Committee of Scottish Parliament's Investigation into Health Impact of GM crops, 14 November 2002 (http://www.gmnews.co.uk/gmnews33.html).

45. Fares, N.H. and El-Sayed, A. K. 1998. Fine structural changes in the ileum of mice fed on dendotoxin-treated potatoes and transgenic potatoes. *Natural Toxins* 6:219–33; also "Bt is toxic" by Joe Cummins and Mae-Wan Ho, *ISIS News* 7/8, February 2001, ISSN: 1474–1547 (print), ISSN: 1474–1814 (online), www.i-sis.org.uk.

46. Pusztai, A. Health impacts of GM crops. Submission of evidence to the Clerk to the Health and Community Care Committee of The Scottish Parliament, 15 Nov 2002 (http://www.gm-news.co.uk/gmnews33.html).

47. Pusztai, A. et al. 1999. Expression of the insecticidal bean alpha-amylase inhibitor transgene has minimal detrimental effect on the nutritional value of peas fed to rats as 30% of the diet. *The Journal of Nutrition* 129:1597–1603.

48. Ewen, S. and Pusztai, A. 1999. Effect of diets containing genetically modified potatoes expressing *Galanthus nivalis* lectin on rat small intestine. *The Lancet* 354:1353–1354; for Pusztai's full rebuttal to his critics, see also http://plab.ku.dk/tcbh/PusztaiPusztai.htm.

49. Pusztai, A. 2002. Can science give us the tools for recognizing possible health risks of GM food? *Nutrition and Health* 16:73–84.

50. Pusztai, A. 2002. GM food safety: Scientific and institutional issues. *Science as Culture* 11:70–92.

51. Pusztai, A., Bardocz, S. and Ewen, S. W. B. 2003. Genetically modified foods: Potential human health effects. In *Food Safety: Contaminants and Toxins*, (J. P. F. D'Mello ed.), Scottish Agricultural College, Edinburgh, CAB International.

52. Vázquez-Padrón, R. I., Moreno-Fierros, L., Neri-Bazán, L., de la Riva, G. and López-Revilla, R. 1999. Intragastric and intraperitoneal administration of Cry1Ac protoxin from *Bacillus thuringiensis* induce systemic and mucosal antibody responses in mice. *Life Sciences* 64:1897–1912.

53. Hernandez, E., Ramisse, F., Cruel, T., le Vagueresse, R. and Cavallo, J. D. 1999. *Bacillus thuringiensis* serotype H34 isolated from human and insecticidal strains serotypes 3a3b and H14 can lead to death of immuno-competent mice after pulmonary infection. *FEMS Immunology and Medical Microbiology* 24:43–47.

54. Cummins, J. Biopesticide and bioweapons. *ISIS Report*, 23 October 2001 (www.i-sis.org.uk).

55. "Poison pharm crops near you" by Joe Cummins, *Science in Society*, 2002, 15; fully referenced version on ISIS members' Web site, www.i-sis.org.uk.

56. Menassa, P., Nguywn, C., Jevnikar, A. and Brindle, J. 2001. A self-contained system for the field production of plant recombinant interleukin-10. *Molecular Breeding* 8:177–185.

57. Cummins, J. Pharming cytokines in transgenic crops. *Science in Society*, 2003, 18, fully referenced version on ISIS members' Web site, www.i-sis.org.uk.

58. Dantzera, R. 2001. Cytokine-induced sickness behavior: Mechanisms and implications. *Annals of the NY Acad. of Sci.* 933:222–234.

59. Bocci, V. 1998. Central nervous system toxicity of interferons and other cytokines. *J. Biol. Regul. Homeost. Agents* 2:107–118.

60. Moulinier, A. 2002. Recombinant interferon alpha induced chorea and subcortical dementia. *Neurology (Correspondence)* 59:18–21.

61. Caracenti, A., Gangeri, L., Martini, C., Belli, F., Brunelli, C., Baldini, M., Mascheroni, L., Lenisa, L. and Cascinetti, N. 1998. Neurotoxicity of interferon alpha in melanoma therapy. *Cancer* 83:482–489.

62. Valentine, A., Meyers, C., Kling, M. A., Richelson, E. and Hauser, P. 1998. Mood and cognitive side effects of interferon alpha. *Semin. Oncol.* 25 (suppl 1):39–47.

63. Ho, M. W. and Cummins, J. SARS and genetic engineering? *ISIS Report*, April 2003; *Science in Society* 18:10–11; fully referenced version on ISIS members' Web site, www.i-sis.org.uk.

64. Tubolya, T., Yub, W., Baileyb, A., Degrandisc, S., Dub, S., Erickson, L. and Nagya, E. Â. 2000. Immunogenicity of porcine transmissible gastroenteritis virus spike protein expressed in plants. *Vaccine* 18:2023–2028.

65. Ho, M. W. Bioterrorism and SARS. *ISIS Report*, April 2003; *Science in Society* 18; fully referenced version on ISIS members' Web site, www.i-sis.org.uk.

66. Prljic, J., Veljkovic, N., Doliana, T., Colombatti, A., Johnson, E., Metlas, R. and Veljkovic, V. 1999. Identification of an active Chi recombinational hot spot within the HIV-1 envelope gene: Consequences for development of AIDS vaccine. *Vaccine* 17:1462–1467.

67. Veljkovic, V. and Ho, M. W. AIDS vaccines or dangerous biological agent? *AIDScience* (http://aidscience.org/Debates/aidscience019d.asp).

68. Ho, M. W. AIDS vaccines trials dangerous. *ISIS News* 11/12, October 2001, ISSN: 1474–1547 (print), ISSN: 1474–1814 (online), www.i-sis.org.uk.

69. Manders, P. and Thomas, R. 2000. Immunology of DNA vaccines: CpG motifs and antigen presentation. *Inflamm. Res.* 49:199–205.

70. Gurunathan, S., Klinman, D. and Seder, R. 2000. DNA Vaccines. *Annu. Rev. Immunol.* 18:927–974.

71. Deng, G., Nilsson, A., Verdrengh, M., Collins, L. and Tarkowski, A. 1999. Intra-articularly located bacteria containing CpG motifs induces arthritis. *Nature Medicine* 5:702–706.

72. Hsu, S., Chung, S., Robertson, D., Ralph, L., Chelvarajan, R. and Bondada, S. 1999. CpG oligodeoxynucleotides rescue BKS-2 immature B cell lymphoma from anti-Ig-M-mediated growth inhibition by up-regulating of egr-1. *International Immunology* 6:871–879.

73. Rui, L., Vinuesa, C. G., Blasioli, J. and Goodnow, C. C. 2003. Resistance to CpG DNA-induced autoimmunity through tolerogenic B cell antigen receptor ERK signalling. *Nature Immunology* 4:594–600.

74. Ho, M. W. and Cummins, J. Chronicle of an ecological disaster foretold. *ISIS Report,* March 2003; fully referenced version on ISIS members' Web site, www.i-sis.org.uk.

75. Hooper, M. Evidence with special emphasis on the use of glufosinate ammonium (phosphinothricin). Chardon LL T25 maize hearing, May 2002; also submitted to the World Health Organization (containing more than 40 references) and posted on ISIS members' Web site, www.i-sis.org.uk.

76. Cummins, J. Glyphosate and glyphosate-tolerant crops. Impacts on health and the environment. *ISIS Report,* June 2002; also submitted to the World Health Organization and posted on ISIS members' Web site, www. i-sis.org.uk; updated April 2003.

77. Canadian Food Inspection Agency Canada Plant Health and Production Division, Plant Biosafety Office 2001, *Decision Document DD95-02: Determination of Environmental Safety of Monsanto Canada Inc.'s Roundup® Herbicide-Tolerant* Brassica napus *Canola Line GT73.*

78. Schonbrunn, E., Eschenburg, S., Shuttleworth, W. A., Schloss, J.V., Amrhein, N., Evans, J. N. S. and Kabsch, W. 2001. Interaction of the herbicide glyphosate with its target enzyme 5-enolpyruvylshikimate 3-phosphate synthase in atomic detail. *PNAS* 98:1376–1380.

79. http://www.pan-uk.orgpestnews/actives/glyphosa.htm, containing many other references.

80. "Weed Killer," *The Progressive,* July 1987 (http://www.natures countrystore.com/roundup/page3.html).

81. Arbuckle, T., Lin, Z. and Mery, L. 2001. An exploratory analysis of the effect of pesticide exposure on the risk of spontaneous abortion in an Ontario farm population. *Envir. Health Perspectives* 109:851–860.

82. Garry, V., Harkins, M., Erickson, L., Long, S., Holland, S. and Burroughs, B. 2002. Birth defects, seasons of conception and sex of children born to pesticide applicators living in the red river valley of Minnesota, USA. *Envir. Health Perspectives* (Suppl. 3) 110:441–449.

83. Dallegrave, E., DiGiorgio, F., Coelho, R., Pereira, J., Dalsenter, P. and Langeloh, A. 2003. The teratogenic potential of the herbicide glyphosate-Roundup in Wistar rats. *Toxicology Letters* 142:45–52.

84. Walsh, L., McCormick, C., Martin, C. and Stocco, D. 2000. Roundup inhibits steroidogenesis by disrupting steroidogenic acute regulatory protein expression. *Envir. Health Perspectives* 108:769–776.

85. Peluso, M., Munnia, A., Bolognisi, C. and Parodi, S. 1998. P32-Post-labeling detection of DNA adducts in mice treated with the herbicide roundup. *Environmental and Mol. Mutagenesis* 31:55–59.

86. Lioi, M., Scarfi, M., Santoro, A., Barbeiri, R., Zeni, O., Barardino, D. and Ursini, M. 1998. Genotoxicity and oxidative stress induced by pesticide exposure in bovine lymphocyte cultures in vitro. *Mut. Res.* 403:13–20.

87. Szarek, J., Siwicki, A., Andrzewska, A., Terech-Majeska, E. and Banaszkiewicz, T. 2000. Effect of the herbicide roundup on the ultrastructural pattern of hepatocytes in carp. *Marine Envir. Res.* 50:263–266.

88. Grisolia, C. 2002. A comparison between mouse and fish micronucleus test using cyclophosphamide, mitomycin C and various pesticides. *Mut. Res.* 400:474, 1–6.

89. Mann, R. and Bidwell, J. 1999. The toxicity of glyphosate and several glyphosate formulations to four species of southwestern Australian frogs. *Archives of Environ. Contam. Toxicol.* 36:193–199.

90. Clements, C., Rapph, S. and Petras, M. Genotoxicity of select herbicides in *Rana catesbeiana* tadpoles using the alkaline single-cell gel DNA electrophoresis (comet) assay. *Env. Mol. Mutagenesis* 29:277–288.

91. Morowati, M. 2000. Histochemical and histopathological study of the intestine of the earthworm exposed to a field dose of the herbicide glyphosate. *The Environmentalist* 20:105–111.

92. Mark, E. J., Lorrilon, O., Boulben, S., Hureau, D., Durrand, G. and Belle, R. 2002. Pesticide roundup provokes cell cycle dysfunction at the level of CDK1/Cyclin B activation. *Chem. Res. Toxicol.* 15:326–331.

93. Ho, M. W. *Living with the Fluid Genome.* ISIS & TWN, London and Penang, 2003, Chapters 8–10.

94. Ho, M. W., Traavik, T., Olsvik, R., Tappeser, B., Howard, V., von Weizsacker, C. and McGavin, G. 1998. Gene Technology and Gene Ecology of Infectious Diseases. *Microbial Ecology in Health and Disease* 10:33–59.

95. Ho, M. W., Ryan, A., Cummins, J. and Traavik, T. *Slipping through the regulatory net. "Naked" and "free" nucleic acids.* TWN Biotechnology & Biosafety Series 5, Third World Network, Penang, 2001.

96. Stemmer, W. P. C. 2002. Molecular breeding of gene, pathways and genomes by DNA shuffling. *Journal of Molecular Catalysis B: Enzymatic* 19–20:2–12.

97. Ho, M. W. 2003. Death by DNA shuffling. *ISIS Report*, April 2003; also *Science in Society* 18: 9 (www.i-sis.org.uk).

98. Ho, M. W., Ryan, A. and Cummins, J. 1999. Cauliflower mosaic viral promoter—A recipe for Disaster? *Microbial Ecology in Health and Disease* 11:194–197.

99. Hodgson, J. 2000. Scientists avert new GMO crisis. *Nature Biotechnology* 18:13.

100. Cummins, J., Ho, M. W. and Ryan, A. 2000. Hazardous CaMV promoter? *Nature Biotechnology* 18:363.

101. Hull, R., Covey, S. N. and Dale, P. 2000. Genetically modified plants and the 35S promoter: Assessing the risks and enhancing the debate. *Microbial Ecology in Health and Disease* 12:1–5.

102. Ho, M. W., Ryan, A. and Cummins, J. 2000. Hazards of transgenic plants with the cauliflower mosaic viral promoter. *Microbial Ecology in Health and Disease* 12:6–11.

103. Courtail, B., Fenebach, F., Ebehard, S., Rhomer, L., Chiapello, H., Carilleri, C. and Lucas, H. 2001. Tnt 1 transposition events are induced by *in vitro* transformation of *Arabidopsis thaliana*, and transposed copies integrated into genes. *Mol. Gen. Genomics* 265:32–42.

104. Ho, M. W., Ryan, A. and Cummins, J. 2000. CaMV35S promoter fragmentation hotspot confirmed and it is active in animals. *Microbial Ecology in Health and Disease* 12:189.

105. The Advisory Committee on Releases to the Environment's (ACRE's) response to concerns raised in written representation and submissions associated with the CHARDON LL public hearing and to statements made at ACRE's open hearing relating to the safety assessment of T25 GM maize conducted under Directive 90/220/EEC (www.defra.gov.uk/ environment/acre).

106. Metz, M. and Futterer, J. Suspect evidence of transgenic contamination. *Nature,* Advance Online Publication, 4 April 2002, www.nature.com; see also Ho, M. W. 2002. Astonishing denial of transgenic pollution. *Science in Society* 15:13–14; fully referenced version on ISIS members' Web site, www.i-sis.org.uk.

107. Bergelson, J., Purrington, C. B. and Wichmann, G. 1998. Promiscuity in transgenic plants. *Nature* 395:25.

108. De Vries, J., and Wackernagel, W. 1998. Detection of nptII (kanamycin resistance) genes in genomes of transgenic plants by marker-rescue transformation. *Mol. Gen. Genet.* 257:606–613.

109. Schluter, K., Futterer, J. and Potrykus, I. 1995. Horizontal gene-transfer from a transgenic potato line to a bacterial pathogen (*Erwinia chrysanthem*) occurs, if at all, at an extremely low frequency. *BioTechnology* 13:1094–1098.

110. Gebhard, F. and Smalla, K. 1999. Monitoring field releases of genetically modified sugar beets for persistence of transgenic plant DNA and horizontal gene transfer. *FEMS Microbiol. Ecol.* 28:261–272.

111. Mercer, D. K., Scott, K. P., Bruce-Johnson, W. A., Glover, L. A. and Flint, H. J. 1999. Fate of free DNA and transformation of the oral bacterium *Streptococcus gordonii* DL1 by plasmid DNA in human saliva. *Applied and Environmental Microbiology* 65:6–10.

112. Duggan, P. S., Chambers, P. A., Heritage, J. and Forbes, J. M. 2000. Survival of free DNA encoding antibiotic resistance from transgenic maize and the transformation activity of DNA in ovine saliva, ovine rumen fluid and silage effluent. *FEMS Microbiology Letters* 191:71–77.

113. Schubbert, R., Rentz, D., Schmitz, B. and Döerfler, W. 1997. Foreign (M13) DNA ingested by mice reaches peripheral leukocytes, spleen and liver via the intestinal wall mucosa and can be covalently linked to mouse DNA. *Proc. Nat. Acad. Sci. USA* 94:961–966.

114. Döerfler, W. and Schubbert, R. 1998. Uptake of foreign DNA from the environment: the gastrointestinal tract and the placenta as portals of entry. *Wien Klin. Wochenschr.* 110:40–44.

115. Traavik, T. 1998. *Too Early May Be Too Late: Ecological Risks Associated with the Use of Naked DNA as a Biological Tool for Research, Production and Therapy.* Report for the Directorate for Nature Research, Trondheim.

116. "Predicted hazards of gene therapy a reality" by Mae-Wan Ho. *ISIS Report*, October 2002 (www.i-sis.org.uk) commenting on *Science*, News of the Week, 4 October 2002; also Ho, M. W. 2003. Gene therapy's first victim. *Science in Society* 17:26–27.

117. Hohlweg, U. and Döerfler, W. 2001. On the fate of plant or other foreign genes upon the uptake in food or after intramuscular injection in mice. *Mol. Genet. Genomics* 265:225–233.

118. Willerslev, E., Hansen, A. J., Binladen, J., Brand, T. B., Gilbert, M. T. P., Shapiro, B., Bunce, M., Winf, C., Gilichinsky, D. A. and Cooper, A. Diverse plant and animal genetic records from Holocene and Pleistocene Sediments. *Sciencexpress Report*, 17 April 2003.

119. "Fears raised over DNA survival in soil," *The Dominion Post* (Wellington), April 25, 2003, via GM Watch (http://www.ngin.org.uk).

120. Netherwood, T., Martin-Orue, S. M., O'Donnell, A. G., Gockling, S., Gilbert, H. J. and Mathers, J. C. *Transgenes in genetically modified Soya survive passage through the small bowel but are completely degraded in the colon.* Technical report on the Food Standards Agency project G010008, "Evaluating the risks associated with using GMOs in human foods," University of Newcastle.

121. Ho, M. W. 2002. Stacking the odds against finding it. *Science in Society* 16:28; fully referenced paper on ISIS members' Web site, www.i-sis.org.uk.

122. Ferguson, G. and Heinemann, J. Recent history of trans-kingdom conjugation. In *Horizontal Gene Transfer*, 2d ed., M. Syvanen and C. I. Kado (eds.). San Diego, Academic Press, 2002.

123. Ho, M. W. 2002. Averting sense for nonsense in horizontal gene transfer. *Science in Society* 16:29–30.

124. McNicol, M. J., Lyon, G. D., Chen, M. Y., Barrett, C. and Cobb, E. 1997. Scottish Crop Research Institute. Contract No RG 0202. The

Possibility of *Agrobacterium* as a Vehicle for Gene Escape. MAFF. *R&D and Surveillance Report: 395.*

125. Cobb, E., MacNicol, R. and Lyon G. 1997. A risk assessment study of plant genetic transformation using *Agrobacterium* and implication for analysis of transgenic plants. *Plant Cell Tissue and Organ Culture* 19:135–144.

126. Kado, C. In *Horizontal Gene Transfer,* 2d ed., M. Syvanen and C. I. Kado (eds.). San Diego, Academic Press, 2002.

127. Sengelov, G., Kristensen, K. J., Sorensen, A. H., Kroer, N. and Sorensen, S. J. 2001. Effect of genomic location on horizontal transfer of a recombinant gene cassette between *Pseudomonas* strains in the rhizosphere and spermosphere of barley seedlings. *Current Microbiology* 42:160–167.

128. Kunik, T., Tzfira, T., Kapulnik, Y., Gafni, Y., Dingwall, C. and Citovsky, V. 2002. Genetic transformation of HeLa cells by *Agrobacterium. PNAS USA* 98:1871–1887; also "Common plant vector injects genes into human cells," *ISIS News* 2002, 11/12, 10, (www.i-sis.org.uk).

129. Ho, M. W. Recent evidence confirms risks of horizontal gene transfer. ISIS' written contribution to ACNFP/Food Standards Agency open meeting 13 November 2002, Cambridge (www.i-sis.org.uk).

130. Pretty, J. and Hine, R. 2001. *Reducing food poverty with sustainable agriculture: A summary of new evidence.* Centre for Environment and Society, Essex University (www2.essex.ac.uk/ces/ResearchProgrammes/CESOccasionalPapers/SAFErepSUBHEADS.htm).

131. Parrott, N. and Marsden, T. 2002. *The real Green Revolution: Organic and agroecological farming in the South.* Greenpeace Environment Trust, London (http://www.greenpeace.org.uk/MultimediaFiles/Live/ FullReport/4526.pdf).

132. Altieri, M. A. *The case against agricultural biotechnology: Why are transgenic crops incompatible with sustainable agriculture in the Third World?* Paper for the NGO briefing packet to the Ministerial Conference and Expo on Agricultural Science and Technology, Sacramento, CA, 2003.

133. *Organic agriculture, environment and food security.* N. E-H. Scialabba and C. Hattam (eds). Rome, Italy, FAO, 2002.

134. Lim, L. C. 2002. Organic agriculture fights back. *Science in Society* 16:30–32.

135. Altieri, M. A., Rosset, P. and Thrupp, L. A. 1998. The potential of agroecology to combat hunger in the developing world (http://www.agroeco.org/fatalharvest/articles/potential_of_agroeco_ch19.pdf).

136. Rosset, P. M. 1999. The multiple functions and benefits of small farm agriculture in the context of global trade negotiations. *Policy Brief No. 4,* Institute for Food and Development Policy (http://www.foodfirst.org/pubs/policybs/pb4.html).

137. "'Magic bean' transforms life for poor Jacks of Central America" by Julian Pettifer, *Independent on Sunday*, 10 June 2001.

138. Kwabiah, A. B., Stoskopf, N. C., Palm, C. A., Voroney, R. P., Rao, M. R. and Gacheru, E. 2003. Phosphorus availability and maize response to organic and inorganic fertilizer inputs in a short term study in western Kenya. *Agriculture, Ecosystems and Environment* 95:49–59.

139. "Get the facts straight: organic agriculture yields are good" by Bill Liebhardt, *Organic Farming Research Foundation Information Bulletin 10*, Summer 2001 (http://www.ofrf.org/publications/news/IB10.pdf).

140. Vasilikiotis, C. 2000. *Can Organic Farming "Feed the World"?* (http://www.agroeco.org/fatalharvest/articles/organic_feed_world.pdf).

141. Petersen, C., Drinkwater, L. E. and Wagoner, P. *The Rodale Institute Farming Systems Trial: The First 15 Years*, The Rodale Institute, 1999.

142. Clark, M. S., Horwath, W. R., Shennan, C., Scow, K. M., Lantni, W. T. and Ferris, H. 1999. Nitrogen, weeds and water as yield-limiting factors in conventional, low-input, and organic tomato systems. *Agriculture, Ecosystems and Environment* 73:257–270.

143. Clark, M. S. et al. 1999. Crop-yield and economic comparisons of organic, low-input, and conventional farming systems in California's Sacramento Valley. *American Journal of Alternative Agriculture* 14(3):109–121; and Clark, M. S. et al. 1998. Changes in soil chemical properties resulting from organic and low-input farming practices. *Agronomy Journal* 90:662–671. Cited in 140.

144. Warman, P. R. and Havard, K. A. 1998. Yield, vitamin and mineral contents of organically and conventionally grown potatoes and sweet corn. *Agriculture, Ecosystems and Environment* 68:207–216.

145. Pearce, F. Desert harvest. *New Scientist*, 27 October 2001, 44–47.

146. Lim, L. C. 2002. Sustainable agriculture pushing back desert. *Science in Society* 15:29.

147. Jenkinson, D. S. et al. In *Long-term experiments in Agricultural and Ecological Sciences*, R. A. Leigh and A. E. Johnston (eds.), p.117–138. CAB International, Wallingford, UK, 1994. Cited in 140.

148. Drinkwater, L. E. et al. 1995. Fundamental differences between conventional and organic tomato agroecosystems in California. *Ecological Applications* 5(4):1098–1112. Cited in 140.

149. Mäder, P., Fliebbach, A., Dubois, D., Gunst, L., Fried, P. and Niggli, U. 2002. Soil fertility and biodiversity in organic farming. *Science* 296:1694–1697.

150. Pearce, F. 20-year study backs organic farming. *New Scientist*, 30 May 2002 (http://www.newscientist.com/news/news.jsp?id=ns99992351).

151. "Soil fungi critical to organic success," USDA Agricultural Research Service, 4 May 2001.

152. Bulluck, III, L. R., Brosius, M., Evanylo, G. K. and Ristaino, J. B. 2002. Organic and synthetic fertility amendments influence soil microbial, physical and chemical properties on organic and conventional farms. *Applied Soil Ecology* 19:147–160.

153. Ryan, A. Organics enter the science wars. *ISIS News* 11/12, October 2001.

154. Drinkwater, L. E., Wagoner, P. and Sarrantonio, M. 1998. Legume-based cropping systems have reduced carbon and nitrogen losses. *Nature* 396:262–265.

155. Tilman, D. 1998. The greening of the green revolution. *Nature* 296:211–212.

156. "100-year drought is no match for organic soybeans," Rodale Institute, 1999 (http://www.rodaleinstitute.org/global/arch_home.html).

157. Poudel, D. D., Horwath, W. R., Lanini, W. T., Temple, S. R. and van Bruggen, A. H. C. 2002. Comparison of soil N availability and leaching potential, crop yields and weeds in organic, low-input and conventional farming systems in northern California. *Agriculture, Ecosystems and Environment* 90:125–137.

158. Oehl, F., Oberson, A., Tagmann, H. U., Besson, J. M., Dubois, D., Mäder, P., Roth, H-R. and Frossard, E. 2002. Phosphorus budget and phosphorus availability in soils under organic and conventional farming. *Nutrient Cycling in Agroecosystems* 62:25–35.

159. Letourneau, D. K. and Goldstein, B. 2001. Pest damage and arthropod community structure in organic vs. conventional tomato production in California. *J. Applied Ecology* 38(3):557–570.

160. Pearce, F. An ordinary miracle. 2001. *New Scientist*, Vol. 169, Issue 2276, p. 16.

161. Barzman, M. and Das, L. 2000. Ecologising rice-based systems in Bangladesh. *ILEIA Newsletter* 16(4):16–17 (http://www.agroeco.org/fatalharvest/articles/ecologising_rice.pdf).

162. "Organic rice is twice as nice" by John Bonner, Report from the International Congress of Ecology, 15 August 2002.

163. Ho, M. W. 1999. One bird—ten thousand treasures. *The Ecologist* 29(6):339–340 and *Third World Resurgence* 1999, 110/111, 2–4.

164. Pimbert, M. Sustaining the multiple functions of agricultural biodiversity. FAO background paper series for the Conference on the Multifunctional Character of Agriculture and Land, The Netherlands, September 1999.

165. *Biodiversity and the ecosystem approach in agriculture, forestry and fisheries*. Proceedings of a satellite event on the occasion of the Ninth Regular Session of the Commission on Genetic Resources for Food and Agriculture, Rome 12-13 October 2002. Rome, Italy, FAO.

166. Scialabba, N. E-H., Grandi, C. and Henatsch, C. Organic agriculture and genetic resources for food and agriculture. In *Biodiversity and the* *ecosystem approach in agriculture, forestry and fisheries*, pp. 72–99. Rome, Italy, FAO, 2002.

167. *Organic agriculture and biodiversity: Making the links.* IFOAM, IUCN and BfN, Germany, 2002; see also Stolton, S. *Organic Agriculture and Biodiversity*, IFOAM Dossier 2, 2002.

168. Azeez, G. *The biodiversity benefits of organic farming*, Soil Association, Bristol, UK, 2000.

169. Burcher, S. 2003. Herbalert to the rescue. *Science in Society* 18:17.

170. Tilman, D., Reich, P. B., Knops, J., Wedin, D., Mielke, T. and Lehman, C. 2001. Diversity and productivity in a long-term grassland experiment. *Science* 294:843–845.

171. Ho, M. W. 2002. Biodiverse systems two to three times more productive than monocultures. *Science in Society* 13/14:36.

172. Zhu, Y., Chen, H., Fan, J., Wang, Y., Li, Y., Chen, J., Fan, J. X., Yang, S., Hu, S., Leung, H., Mew, T. W., Teng, P. S., Wang, Z. and Mundt, C. 2000. Genetic diversity and disease control in rice. *Nature* 406:718–722.

173. "Simple Method Found to Vastly Increase Crop Yields" by Carol Kaesuk Yoon, *New York Times*, 22 August 2000.

174. Bennack, D., Brown, G., Bunning, S. and de Cunha, M. H. 2002. Soil biodiversity management for sustainable and productive agriculture: Lessons from case studies. In *Biodiversity and the ecosystem approach in agriculture, forestry and fisheries*, pp.196–223, FAO.

175. Reganold, J. P., Glover, J. D., Andrews, P. K. and Hinman, J. R. 2001. Sustainability of three apple production systems. *Nature* 410:926–930.

176. "Organic apples win productivity and taste trials," 10 August 2001, Pesticide Action Network Updates Service (http://www.panna.org).

177. Pacini, C., Wossink, A., Giesen, G., Vazzana, C. and Huirne, R. 2003. Evaluation of sustainability of organic, integrated and conventional farming systems: a farm and field-scale analysis. *Agriculture, Ecosystems and Environment* 95:273–288.

178. Stolze, M., Piorr, A., Häring, A. and Dabbert, S. *Environmental and resource use impacts of organic farming in Europe*, Commission of the European Communities, Agriculture and Fisheries (FAIR) specific RTD program, Fair3-CT96-1794, "Effects of the CAP-reform and possible further development on organic farming in the EU," 1999.

179. Goldsmith, E. How to feed people under a regime of climate change (unpublished paper), 2003.

180. Lötjönen T. 2003. Machine work and energy consumption in organic farming. *Ecology and Farming* 32:7–8, IFOAM.

181. Dalgaard T. 2003. On-farm fossil energy use. *Ecology and Farming* 32:9, IFOAM.

182. Porter, P. M., Huggins, D. R., Perillo, C. A., Quiring, S. R. and Crookston, R. K. 2003. Organic and other management strategies with two- and four-year crop rotations in Minnesota. *Agronomy Journal* 95(2):233–244.

183. Welsh, R. 1999. *The Economics of Organic Grain and Soybean Production in the Midwestern United States.* Henry A. Wallace Institute for Alternative Agriculture (http://www.agroeco.org/fatalharvest/articles/economics_organic_prod.pdf).

184. Rosset, P. "Taking seriously the claim that genetic engineering could end hunger: A critical analysis," pp. 81–93 in Britt Bailey and Marc Lappé (eds), *Engineering the Farm: Ethical and Social Aspects of Agricultural Biotechnology.* Washington, DC, Island Press, 2002.

185. Chambers, R., Pacey, A. and Thrupp, L. A. 1989. *Farmer First: Farmer Innovation and Agriculture Research,* Intermediate Technology Publications, London, UK.

186. Scoones, I. and Thompson, J. 1994. *Beyond Farmer First: Rural People's Knowledge, Agricultural Research and Extension Practice,* Intermediate Technology Publications, London, UK.

187. *Agroecological Innovations: Increasing Food Production with Participatory Development,* Norman Uphoff (ed.). Earthscan Publications, 2002.

188. Lim, L. C. 2003. Ethiopia's own agriculture. *Science in Society* 17:7–8.

189. Uphoff, N. and Altieri, M. A. 1999. *Alternatives to conventional modern agriculture for meeting world food needs in the next century.* (Report of a Conference "Sustainable Agriculture: Evaluation of New Paradigms and Old Practices", Bellagio, Italy). Cornell International Institute for Food, Agriculture, and Development, Ithaca, NY. Cited in ref. 4.

190. Pretty, J. 1995. *Regenerating agriculture.* Earthscan, London, UK. Cited in ref. 4.

191. Rundgren, G. *Organic Agriculture and Food Security,* IFOAM Dossier 1, 2002.

192. Boyde, T. *Cusgarne Organics local money flows.* New Economics Foundation and The Countryside Agency, London, 2001.

193. Heaton, S. 2001. *Organic farming, food quality and human health: A review of the evidence.* Soil Association, Bristol, UK.

194. Tielemans, E., van Kooij, E., te Velde, E. R., Burdorf, A. and Heederik, D. 1999. Pesticide exposure and decreased fertilisation rates in vitro. *The Lancet* 354:484–485.

195. Abell, A., Ersnt, E. and Bonde, J. P. 1994. High sperm density among members of organic farmers' association. *The Lancet* 343:1498.

196. Jensen, T. K., Giwercman, A., Carlsen, E., Scheike, T. and Skakkebaek, N. E. 1996. Semen quality among members of organic food associations in Zealand, Denmark. *The Lancet* 347:1844.

197. Curl, C. L., Fenske, R. A. and Elgethun, K. 2003. Organophosphorus pesticide exposure of urban and suburban preschool children with organic and conventional diets. *Environmental Health Perspectives* 111(3):377–382.

198. Worthington, V. 2001. Nutritional quality of organic versus conventional fruits, vegetables, and grains. *The Journal of Alternative and Complementary Medicine* 7(2):161–173.

199. Asami, D. K., Hong, Y. J., Barrett, D. M. and Mitchell, A. E. 2003. Comparison of the total phenolic and ascorbic acid content of freeze-dried and air-dried marionberry, strawberry, and corn grown using conventional, organic, and sustainable agricultural practices. *J. Agric. Food Chem.* 51(5):1237–1241, 10.1021/jf020635c S0021-8561.

200. Cummins, J. Organic agriculture helps fight cancer. *ISIS Report*, 27 March 2003 (www.i-sis.org.uk).

201. Carbonaro, M., Mattera, M., Nicoli, S., Bergamo, P. and Cappelloni, M. 2002. Modulation of antioxidant compounds in organic vs conventional fruit (Peach, *Prunus persica* L., and Pear, *Pyrus communis* L.). *J. Agric. Food Chem.* 50:5458–5462.

202. Novotny, E. 2002. Report IV—The Wheel of Health (in the Chardon LL T25 maize hearing listings) (http://www.sgr.org.uk/GMOs.html).

203. Novotny, E. 2003. Letter to MSPs on the Organic Farming Targets Bill (http://www.sgr.org.uk/GMOs.html).

Statement of the Independent Science Panel
Launched 10 May 2003, London

The Independent Science Panel (ISP) is a panel of scientists from many disciplines, committed to the following.

1. **Promoting science for the public good, independent of commercial and other special interests, or of government control.**

We firmly believe that science should be accountable to civil society; that it should be accessible to all, regardless of gender, age, race, religion or caste; and that all sectors of civil society should participate in making decisions on all issues related to science, from scientific research to policies regarding science and technologies.

We believe that accurate scientific information should be promptly accessible to the public in unbiased and uncensored forms.

2. **Maintaining the highest standards of integrity and impartiality in science.**

We subscribe to the principles of honesty, openness and pluralism in the practice of science. There should be open peer-review for published work, and respect and protection for those whose research challenges the conventional paradigm or majority opinion. Scientific disagreements must be openly and democratically debated.

We are committed to upholding the highest standards of scientific research, and to ensuring that research funding is not skewed or distorted by commercial or political imperatives.

3. **Developing sciences that can help make the world sustainable, equitable, peaceful and life-enhancing for all its inhabitants.**

We respect the sanctity of human life, seek to minimize harm to any living creature, and protect the environment. We hold that science should contribute to the physical, social and spiritual well-being of all in all societies.

We are committed to an ecological perspective that takes proper account of the complexity, diversity and interdependence of all nature.

We subscribe to the precautionary principle: when there is reasonable suspicion of serious or irreversible damage, lack of scientific consensus must not be used to postpone preventative action.

We reject scientific endeavors that serve aggressive military ends, promote commercial imperialism or damage social justice.

The Genetic Modification Group of the ISP

The Genetic Modification (GM) Group of the ISP consists of scientists working in genetics, biosciences, toxicology and medicine, and other representatives of civil society who are concerned about the harmful consequences of genetic modifications of plants and animals and related technologies and their rapid commercialization in agriculture and medicine without due process of proper scientific assessment and of public consultation and consent.

We find the following aspects especially regrettable and unacceptable:

- Lack of critical public information on the science and technology of GM
- Lack of public accountability in the GM science community
- Lack of independent, disinterested scientific research into, and assessment of, the hazards of GM
- Partisan attitude of regulatory and other public information bodies, which appear more intent on spreading corporate propaganda than providing crucial information
- Pervasive commercial and political conflicts of interests in both research and development and regulation of GM
- Suppression and vilification of scientists who try to convey research information to the public that is deemed to harm the industry
- Persistent denial and dismissal of extensive scientific evidence on the hazards of GM to health and the environment by proponents of genetic modification and by supposedly disinterested advisory and regulatory bodies

- Continuing claims of GM benefits by the biotech corporations, and repetitions of these claims by the scientific establishment, in the face of extensive evidence that GM has failed both in the field and in the laboratory.
- Reluctance to recognize that the corporate funding of academic research in GM is already in decline, and that the biotechnology multinationals (and their shareholders) as well as investment consultants are now questioning the wisdom of the "GM enterprise"
- Attacks on, and summary dismissal of, extensive evidence pointing to the benefits of various sustainable agricultural approaches for health and the environment, as well as for food security and social well-being of farmers and their local communities.

Independent Science Panel on GM
List of Members

Prof. Miguel Altieri
Professor of Agroecology, University of California, Berkeley, USA

Dr. Michael Antoniou
Senior Lecturer in Molecular Genetics, GKT School of Medicine, King's College, London

Dr. Susan Bardocz
Biochemist; formerly Rowett Research Institute, Scotland

Prof. David Bellamy OBE
Internationally renowned botanist, environmentalist, broadcaster, author and campaigner; recipient of numerous awards; president and vice president of many conservation and environmental organizations

Dr. Elizabeth Bravo V.
Biologist, researcher and campaigner on biodiversity and GMO issues; cofounder of Acción Ecológica; part-time lecturer at Universidad Politécnica Salesiana, Ecuador

Prof. Joe Cummins
Professor Emeritus of Genetics, University of Western Ontario, London, Ontario, Canada

Dr. Stanley Ewen
Consultant histopathologist at Grampian University Hospitals Trust; formerly senior lecturer in pathology, University of Aberdeen; lead histopathologist for the Grampian arm of the Scottish Colorectal Cancer Screening Pilot Project

Edward Goldsmith
Recipient of the Right Livelihood and numerous awards, environmentalist, scholar, author and founding editor of *The Ecologist*

Dr. Brian Goodwin
Scholar in Residence, Schumacher College, England

Dr. Mae-Wan Ho
Cofounder and Director of the Institute of Science in Society; Editor of the magazine *Science in Society*; science advisor to the Third World Network and on the Roster of Experts for the Cartagena Protocol on Biosafety

Prof. Malcolm Hooper
Emeritus Professor at the University of Sunderland; previously, Professor of Medicinal Chemistry, faculty of Pharmaceutical Sciences, Sunderland Polytechnic; chief scientific advisor to the Gulf War Veterans

Dr. Vyvyan Howard
Medically qualified toxico-pathologist, Developmental Toxico-Pathology Group, Department of Human Anatomy and Cell Biology, The University of Liverpool; member of the UK Government's Advisory Committee on Pesticides

Dr. Brian John
Geomorphologist and environmental scientist; founder and long-time chairman of the West Wales Eco Centre; one of the coordinating group of GM Free Cymru

Prof. Marijan Joπt
Professor of Plant Breeding and Seed Production, Agricultural College Krizevci, Croatia

Lim Li Ching
Researcher, Institute of Science in Society and Third World Network; deputy-editor of *Science in Society* magazine

Dr. Eva Novotny
Astronomer and campaigner on GM issues for Scientists for Global Responsibility (SGR)

Prof. Bob Orskov OBE
Formerly Rowett Research Institute, Aberdeen, Scotland; Director, International Feed Resources Unit; Fellow of the Royal Society of Edinburgh (FRSE); Fellow of the Polish Academy of Science

Dr. Michel Pimbert
Agricultural ecologist and Principal Associate, International Institute for Environment and Development

Dr. Arpad Pusztai
Private consultant; formerly Senior Research Fellow at the Rowett Research Institute, Bucksburn, Aberdeen, Scotland

David Quist
Microbial ecologist, Ecosystem Sciences Division, Environmental Science, Policy and Management, University of California, Berkeley, USA

Dr. Peter Rosset
Agricultural ecologist and rural development specialist; Codirector of the Institute for Food and Development Policy (Food First), Oakland, California, USA

Prof. Peter Saunders
Professor of Applied Mathematics at King's College, London

Dr. Veljko Veljkovic
AIDS virologist, Center for Multidisciplinary Research and Engineering, Institute of Nuclear Sciences VINCA, Belgrade, Yugoslavia

Prof. Oscar B. Zamora
Professor of Agronomy, Department of Agronomy, University of the Philippines Los Banos-College of Agriculture (UPLB-CA), College, Laguna, The Philippines

Independent Science Panel Web site: www.indsp.org

Index

US GM/Sustainable Resources

Acres USA: www.acresusa.com (Phone: 1-800-355-5313)
Alliance for Sustainability: www.allianceforsustainability.net
   (Phone: 1-612-331-1099)
The Campaign to Label Genetically Engineered Food:
   www.thecampaign.org (Phone: 1-425-771-4049)
Center for Ethics and Toxics: www.cetos.org
   (Phone: 1-707-884-1700)
The Center for Food Safety: www.centerforfoodsafety.org
   (Phone: 1-202-547-9359)
Citizens for Health: www.citizens.org (Phone: 1-202-483-4344)
Consumer's Choice Council: www.consumerscouncil.org
   (Phone: 1-202-785-1950)
CorpWatch: www.corpwatch.org (Phone: 1-510-271-8080)
Food First: www.foodfirst.org (Phone: 1-510-654-4400)
GE Food Alert Coalition: www.gefoodalert.org
Greenpeace True Food Network: www.truefoodnow.org
   (Phone: 1-415-512-9024)
Institute for Agriculture and Trade Policy: www.iatp.org
   (Phone: 1-612-870-0453)
Organic Trade Association: www.ota.com (Phone: 1-413-774-7511)
Organic Consumer's Association: www.organicconsumers.org
   (Phone: 1-218-226-4164)
The Rodale Institute: www.thenewfarm.org (Phone: 1-610-683-1408)
Sierra Club, US: www.sierraclub.org/biotech
   (Phone: 1-415-977-5500)
State Public Interest Resource Groups: www.pirg.org

International GM/Sustainable Resources

Australia:
Network of Concerned Farmers: www.non-gm-farmers.com
   (Phone: 02-6672-8373)
Organic Federation of Australia: www.ofa.org.au
   (Phone: 08-8370-8455)

Canada:
Convention on Biological Diversity: www.biodiv.org
   (Phone: 1-514-287 7030)

National Farmers Union: www.nfu.ca (Phone: 1-306-652-9465)
Sierra Club Canada: www.sierraclub.ca (Phone: 1-613-241-4611)

France:
Ecosens: www.ecosens.org

Multinational:
Consumers International: www.consumersinternational.org
  (Phone: 011-44-207-226-6663)
Greenpeace International (Browse by nation):
  www.greenpeace.org (Phone: 011-31-20-523-62-22)
International Federation of Organic Agriculture Movements:
  www.ifoam.org (Phone: 011-49-6853-919890)
Northern Alliance for Sustainability: www.anped.org
  (Phone: 011-31-20-4751742)
Third World Network: www.twnside.org.sg
  (Phone: 011-60-4-2266728)
European NGO-Network on Genetic Engineering:
  www.genet-info.org (Phone: 011-49-531-5168746)

New Zealand:
Mothers Against Genetic Engineering: www.madge.net.nz
  (Phone: 09-309-38-38)

Spain:
Genetic Resources Action International: www.grain.org
  (Phone: 34-933011381)

Switzerland:
Bioterra: www.bioterra.ch (Phone: 1-463-55-14)

UK:
Friends of the Earth: www.foe.co.uk (Phone: 020-7490-1555)
Genewatch UK: www.genewatch.org
GM Food News: www.gmfoodnews.com
The Institute of Science in Society: www.i-sis.org.uk
  (Phone: 020-8643-0681)
Soil Association: www.soilassociation.org (Phone: 0117-929-0661)
Sustain: www.sustainweb.org (Phone: 020 7837 1228)
UK Agricultural Biodiversity Coalition: www.ukfg.org.uk

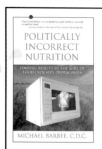
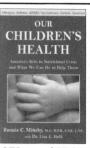
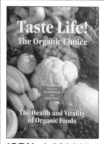
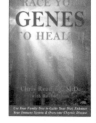